The Birth of Acupuncture in America

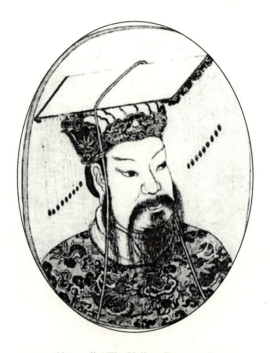

Huangdi, "The Yellow Emperor,"
the legendary founder of Chinese civilization

The Birth of Acupuncture in America

The White Crane's Gift

Steven Rosenblatt, MD, PhD, L.Ac
&
Keith Kirts

Copyright © 2016 Steven Rosenblatt and Keith Kirts

All rights reserved. No part of this book may be used or reproduced by any means, graphic, electronic, or mechanical, including photocopying, recording, taping or by any information storage retrieval system without the written permission of the author except in the case of brief quotations embodied in critical articles and reviews.

Book design by Pablo Capra
Cover design by Kathleen Rosenblatt

Balboa Press books may be ordered through booksellers or by contacting:

Balboa Press
A Division of Hay House
1663 Liberty Drive
Bloomington, IN 47403
www.balboapress.com
1 (877) 407-4847

Because of the dynamic nature of the Internet, any web addresses or links contained in this book may have changed since publication and may no longer be valid. The views expressed in this work are solely those of the author and do not necessarily reflect the views of the publisher, and the publisher hereby disclaims any responsibility for them.

The author of this book does not dispense medical advice or prescribe the use of any technique as a form of treatment for physical, emotional, or medical problems without the advice of a physician, either directly or indirectly. The intent of the author is only to offer information of a general nature to help you in your quest for emotional and spiritual well-being. In the event you use any of the information in this book for yourself, which is your constitutional right, the author and the publisher assume no responsibility for your actions.

Any people depicted in stock imagery provided by Thinkstock are models,
and such images are being used for illustrative purposes only.
Certain stock imagery © Thinkstock.

Print information available on the last page.

ISBN: 978-1-5043-6431-7 (sc)
ISBN: 978-1-5043-6433-1 (hc)
ISBN: 978-1-5043-6432-4 (e)

Library of Congress Control Number: 2016914333

Balboa Press rev. date: 09/06/2016

DEDICATION

To our teachers,
who took what little we gave, and gave what could never be taken away.

To our fellow travelers,
warriors on the path, who knowingly or sometimes unknowingly aided, inspired and supported us.

To our children and students,
who continue this journey of unfolding discovery.

ACKNOWLEDGMENTS

Kathleen Rosenblatt
for editorial assistance and cover design.

Dan Cytron
for computer input: faci@flash.net

Contents

Introduction 9
Prologue 11

CHAPTER ONE
    Talks on the Malibu Pier 14

CHAPTER TWO
    Energy at Birth 27

CHAPTER THREE
    Energetics 39

CHAPTER FOUR
    Energetics 2A 59

CHAPTER FIVE
    Techniques in Gwa Sah & Moxa 67

CHAPTER SIX
    Five Aspects of Energy 75

CHAPTER SEVEN
    The Yellow Emperor, and More 84

CHAPTER EIGHT
    First-Aid with Acupuncture 92

CHAPTER NINE
    Layers of Disease 98

CHAPTER TEN
    Causes of Disease 102

SECTION 2
THE PRACTICE

CHAPTER ELEVEN
    Techniques for Diagnosis 108

CHAPTER TWELVE
    Homeopathy 114

CHAPTER THIRTEEN
    A Diet for 21st Century Foxes 121

CHAPTER FOURTEEN
    Herbal First Aid and Dr. Ju's Arrest 128

CHAPTER FIFTEEN
    First Aid Massage 138

CHAPTER SIXTEEN
    Riding the Tiger.. 143

About the Authors 157

Introduction

Acupuncture for North Americans first blossomed in Los Angeles, downtown in Chinatown.

The year was 1968—a magical time. Everyone felt it. To be alive in the late Sixties was to be part of The Beatles, Bob Dylan, the Love-ins, Viet Nam protests, and Civil Rights marches. Even down in Chinatown, where Dr. Ju, Gim Shek had lived for ten years since coming from Hong Kong, there was quiet excitement in the air.

Many new things were being born into the world. Among the births was the American Acupuncture Movement, which breathed its first breath at Dr. Ju's apartment near Dodger Stadium.

Dr. Ju, or as his students called him, Dr. Kim, was almost single-handedly responsible for the development of acupuncture in the United States. His willingness to adopt a group of UCLA graduate students to train in the ancient medical arts was an unprecedented break from Chinese tradition—inspired by his vision for a better world.

As Dr. Ju often lamented, acupuncture was reaching a low point in China. He sought to graft it onto the vitality of the Western culture. The West, with all its problems, would be the new flowering of acupuncture and related healing techniques. California was the perfect fertile soil for the growth of this new ancient medicine.

Here for the first time we are presenting excerpts of his collected thoughts in a journal format. Dr. Ju's Journal is a literary device which we developed to give a personal voice to his vision and ideas. It is formed of oral transmissions directly from Dr. Ju himself, as well as collected reflections from his colleagues such as Dr. So, Tin Yau and Marshall Ho'o, from his daughters, and from his other Chinese students such as Howard Lee. These journal entries provide an insight into Dr. Ju's personal mission and his methods of transmitting this ancient knowledge.

For thousands of years, the white crane has been the symbol of the doctor in Taoist China. The myth of the flying stork (a type of white crane) bringing the newborn baby is a European adaptation of the Chinese symbolism. To his students, Dr. Ju, Gim Shek was the embodiment of the white crane, the doctor. Acupuncture in America is truly a gift from the storehouse of ancient Chinese knowledge. It is the White Crane's gift.

* * *

Prologue

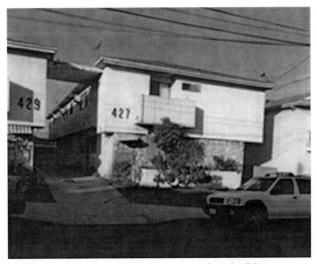

Dr. Ju's apartment in Chinatown... where it all began.

Dr. Steven Rosenblatt has been riding the back of the tiger known as the American Acupuncture Movement since the moment it was born. Along with Bill Prensky and Louie Prince, Steve and his soon to be wife, Kathleen Ferrick, became the first students of Dr. Ju Gim Shek, a respected acupuncturist living in LA's Chinatown, who had been forced to flee from mainland China due to the Maoist revolution some years earlier.

Rosenblatt and Prensky were graduate lab partners at UCLA's Department of Psychology, studying brain chemistry and the mechanisms of pain. The lure of an ancient way of dealing with pain drew them like a magnet to Chinatown. The magic carpet of Chinese medicine was waiting there to unroll for them. Since the fateful meeting with Dr. Ju in 1968, every day of their lives has been involved with bringing this non-invasive medicine to the West. Even a casual glance at how many acupuncturists there are today shows that their success has been astounding.

In 1972, Prensky, Rosenblatt and Dr. Ju, along with David Bresler, another lab partner at UCLA, started the National Acupuncture Association. This small organization was instrumental in passing the first acupuncture licensing legislation in California, Nevada and Oregon. They founded the first acupuncture clinic in the United States in a third floor wing of the UCLA Psychology Building.

The tiger of acupuncture is still running strongly and Dr. Steve Rosenblatt is still riding and hanging on tightly. This book is the story of that ride.

*

Dr. Rosenblatt and I are friends. We first met at a tai-chi class in the early Seventies and we clicked. Since then we have spent thousands of hours together as tennis buddies, going to baseball games, and becoming semi-connoisseurs of Japanese sushi and sake. We even became fishing buddies after deciding to introduce our young daughters to the mysteries of nature and the outdoors by taking them fishing, even though neither of us knew enough about fishing to put into a thimble. In short, we have done most of the male bonding rituals that our culture provides.

But the real bond between us occurred because we have been meeting once a week over a rather long number of years to jot down and organize notes on this amazing event that we have both been part of—the birth of acupuncture in America.

Seemingly by accident, I have become a witness to much of the American Acupuncture Movement. It has been an interesting and almost effortless role to fill, but now that we are organizing this rather vast body of notes into a book, I wish that I had paid even better attention. Already things and people are disappearing into the mists of history, and it wasn't even that long ago. We have decided not to write an exhaustive history; but we are presenting historical notes and stories centered around Dr. Ju and Dr. Rosenblatt, because that's what we know best. We're also going to highlight Dr. Rosenblatt's views on Energetic Medicine, including acupuncture and homeopathy, proven by 40 years on the front lines of medical practice *doing the doctor* as Dr. Ju was fond of saying.

The all-time best-selling book on acupuncture and Chinese medicine is *The Yellow Emperor's Classic on Chinese Medicine..* This book has been selling steadily since at least two centuries before Christ was born. One of the reasons is the Question & Answer format between an enlightened simpleton, The Yellow Emperor, and Li Po, his court acupuncturist. Hoping for a similar longevity, we are also going to use the Q & A style—with me playing the part of the simpleton, a role which has always been easy for me.

* * *

Chapter One

Talks on the Malibu Pier

"When you ride the tiger, be sure to hold on tight."
Old Chinese saying

The girls were running up and down the wooden planking of the Malibu Pier, already tired of not catching any fish. Dr. Rosenblatt and I were leaning on the wooden railing, watching our bait soaking in the blue/green waves rolling endlessly against the wooden pilings on their way to the beach.

"What's the most important thing about acupuncture?" I asked, taking my role as Scribe seriously. The time had come. We were off and running on the book. This was the first of several million questions that I was prepared to ask.

"The central idea of acupuncture," Dr. Rosenblatt answered without hesitation, "is the study of energy in the human body. If even one-tenth of the people in this country could grasp the concept of Energetics, everything would be different. Everything."

"You mean medicine...?" I inquired, supposing that's what he meant.

"All kinds of things, including health and medicine. We wouldn't buy food with additives and pesticides. Farming and commerce would have to stop using lethal poisons. As we started feeling better, we'd relate to each other differently. It would be a very healthy change.

"For instance, take the idea that the physical body *wants* to be in a state of perfect health, and is trying all the time to promote this perfect state for itself. Medicine should assist this effort of the body. It's becoming more and more evident to me that the secret of effective medical treatment is through a study of the energy that courses through all of us. Energy, actually, is the life force that animates all living beings."

Chapter One

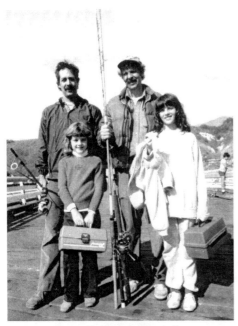

Steve, Keith and girls at pier
PHOTO: Kathleen Rosenblatt

"That's fairly evident," I said, twiddling my pen in the air.

"Perhaps evident to you," he said, "but not to many people."

"You mean I've been hanging around with you so long that thinking of flowing energy seems normal to me?"

He laughed. "I guess so. All living things are energy beings, formed on an energetic pattern. Bio-electric energy flowing along pathways (acupuncture meridians) in the body creates a bio-magnetic life-force. This energy animates all the functions of the body. Alterations in the energy produce a condition known as disease. Evenly flowing, balanced energy produces health. The Chinese call this energy *Chi*, the Japanese call it *Ki*.

"Energetic medicine seeks to understand and manipulate this flow of energy. While Western medicine deals mostly with diseased organisms, energetic medicine focuses on the underlying energy that fills the body with life.

"Let me give you a simple example of energy. Take a magnet, the kind that everybody knows about—the kind stuck on the door of your refrigerator holding the grocery list. Every magnet has an energy field around it. This energy field exerts its force through the air. It doesn't have wires—but held a few inches from an iron object, it will attract the iron."

"Almost like magic," I said.

"This magnetic field can be made visible by using of a handful of iron dust. The magnet attracts the dust and reveals the energy field."

"Magnetism is one kind of energy—and we are discovering that magnetic energy has healing properties. It also is a model for the body's energy.

"In the same way that the magnet has fields of energy, the body has the same kind of energy lines—we call them the acupuncture meridians. However, if we drop our refrigerator magnet on the sidewalk a few times, its

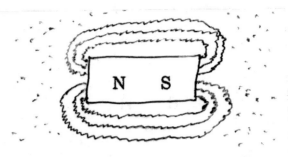

Magnet Attracting Iron Dust

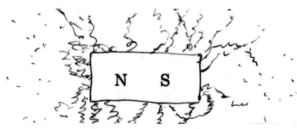

Tangled (Damaged) Energy Lines

energy field gets damaged and the lines become tangled or jumbled."

"This same condition of tangling happens to the energy lines in our bodies due to daily stress, toxins in modern cities and the unhealthy fast food we eat."

"Sounds perfectly reasonable to me," I said. "Sometimes I feel tangled and jangled. Why didn't I learn this stuff about magnets and human energetic in high school?"

"Hopefully our grandchildren will." He smiled, ruefully.

*

Dr. Ju's Journal—1—Autumn, 1968

For many years I had been doing a daily walking meditation in the large park near my apartment in Chinatown. Suddenly several Anglo boys joined the t'ai chi class in my park—a thing that had never happened before, not ever in recorded history that I knew of. I watched them occasionally from afar, even stopping my walking to watch. It piqued my curiosity—and more than that, an echo formed in my mind—something forgotten was nagging at me—a task still to be accomplished. Many years ago, the old Taoist monks at my monastery in Canton Province had suggested that I should bring acupuncture to America. And I had agreed to follow their suggestion by migrating—but as I observed the t'ai chi practice, a cloudy memory of what they really meant began reemerging.

After riding over on the ocean liner ship with my few belongings, I had set up medical practice in a stucco flat on a side street of Chinatown, Los Angeles, within walking distance of my favorite restaurants, my men's club and this park. I treated many people with traditional Taoist medicine—acupuncture and Chinese herbs. But only Chinese people came for cures, not white barbarians—in such a hurry with their penicillin, pills and surgery.

Four times a week, these young medical fellows from the Brain Research Department at UCLA were practicing t'ai chi chuan with Marshall Ho'o's class. Had the monks meant that I was preordained to disseminate the curing arts using these America boys? It seemed that my friend, Marshall Ho'o had rounded them up for just this purpose. Hmmm. That thought had some teeth in it.

Pursuing cautiously, I got myself invited to the public t'ai chi demonstration that Marshall was presenting as part of the Chinese New Year's celebration. Oddly, it was the American boys that were demonstrating t'ai chi up on stage under the pagoda while the Chinese students performed some type of baton twirling—what a strange mixing of cultures.

I approached cautiously, but boldly, for the signs and portents that I had forgotten were suddenly very present. These UCLA students were somewhat serious. They practiced. I could tell by watching. But were they the ones in my dream vision or not?

Then, on the very first introduction, after the fine demonstration, Marshall somehow garbled my proud family name. The UCLA boys thought he said Kim instead of Gim, so they jubilantly named me Dr. Kim and began treating me like their new best buddy. A Chinese doctor as a buddy? That was not a correct way to treat a teacher, at all.

And in spite of this, I found myself inviting them to visit my home. Fate was singing very strongly in my left ear. Correctness was everywhere. Inviting white strangers to my house. Unheard of...! Barbarian college boys? Well, did it matter, really, that they weren't aware enough to call me by my real name? One can't expect much from Lo-fan? These were the ones that I was going to teach, with their inflated egos and happy smiles. The omens were very clear.

*

"Have you ever thought about the Earth?" Dr. Rosenblatt asked, gazing at the coastline, which stretched all the way around the Santa Monica Bay from Malibu south to Palos Verdes like a Chinese landscape under a very cloudy sky.

"What about the Earth?" I asked.

"Well, it's like a big ball-magnet with invisible lines similar to magnetic field lines—also similar to the body's acupuncture meridians."

"Lines of energy," I said, picking up on his thought.

"Not quite," the Doc said. "More like fields of energy. A line only has one dimension; but the Earth is very three dimensional—so we must get used to viewing energy as force rather than as a line. We're like a fish in water—we swim through the Earth's magnetic field, just like a fish swims along a current of warm water."

"Interesting," I said, somewhat astonished that such a simple concept could have eluded me my whole life.

"Yes. They're starting to think that migratory birds orient themselves with this grid of magnetic energy."

"I thought nobody knew how homing pigeons could find their way home."

"Well, they don't know exactly, but researchers are fixing magnets to a bird, and it seems to confuse their sense of direction."

"Hmmm," I said, noticing that a ragged blue/gray rain cloud was blowing across the sky right at us. It was definitely going to rain. "Maybe we should buy a fish at the market to take home."

"Fresh fish make happy face," he quoted. "That's what Dr. Ju used to say every time we went out for fish—and every time a fish dish arrived at the table." The Doc smiled, evidently remembering the fish he'd eaten with Dr. Ju. "Fresh fish make happy face," he repeated.

*

Dr. Ju's Journal—2—Winter, 1968

One morning, the UCLA boys came over and knocked on my apartment door. What could I do? I had invited them. They came. Now I had to teach them. So my second life mission could finally start, now that I had remembered it. I was so happy inside that I said a little prayer of thanksgiving to Lao Tsu,

CHAPTER ONE

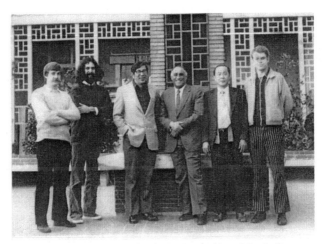

Dr. Tymowski's assistant, Dr. Rosenblatt, Marshall Ho'o, Dr. J. C. de Tymowski, Dr. Ju, Louie Prince

something I had never done before.

It's no fun to be a cultured person stuck in a foreign country where all your skills and subtleties are discounted. Well, I have had some fun here; but it is very fine that the mission is finally starting, so I can go home someday to find peace and serenity.

Really, I couldn't get over my good luck. They were just like the vision that Ancestor Lu showed me in the dream so long ago back in China. The Politico, Bill, bright and dedicated, wearing steel-rimmed glasses. Louie, the unhappy Mystic, lost in dreams. And Steve, the Man of Action, the Chairman, undeterred by hardships. The Chairman's dark-haired Anglo wife was missing. The vision clearly showed her with him; but evidently she would be along later. My heart was beating with happiness and awe.

My little group, knocking on my door. So adventuresome, so brash. Nice boys. I was well pleased. And just in the nick of time to meet Tymowski, the Frenchman, who was arriving next month to spread the gospel of the International Association of Acupuncture. An International Association, well why not? I was sure that my new students were very credible, and credentialed. Brain students from UCLA. Marshall Ho'o had said so.

And then I heard another odd circumstance. The son of old Master Tung, Fu Ling, Marshall Ho'o's T'ai Chi teacher, was coming to Los Angeles to set up a T'ai Chi studio. Everyone said that young Tung was extraordinary. This was very synchronous. Very surprising. These smiling young UCLA fellows were going to be very fortunate at their Five Excellences.

But they all need a haircut. How can I be seen around town with them looking like that?

*

"So if we're swimming in a sea of magnetic energy, inside and outside," I said, after making sure that the girls were still in sight, "you'd think that nobody would get sick. Isn't magnetic energy supposed to be good for people?"

"Yes, but it's a little more complicated than that," Dr. R said, pulling a pen out of his pocket. "Thanks to the layer of organic life on the Earth's surface (trees, the soil, birds, humans) we're living in a bio-energetic hot-house. Bio-magnetic energy is the stuff of life.

"Regular magnetic energy and the electricity that lights a light bulb is bi-polar (two poles, North and South). Bio-energy, on the other hand, is tri-polar like the Yin/Yang diagram." With the ball-point pen, he drew a diagram on the railing. The next guy who fished from this spot would probably wonder about that. Maybe he'd think it was a diagram for a new fishing theory.

Yin/Yang

"Yin/Yang has North and South poles, and it also contains a very subtle 3rd force, which Dr. Ju explained as the *Tao*. The S shaped line that defines the light and dark forces is an element in its own right. Look at it. It even looks energetic." He squiggled another diagram.

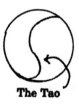

The Tao

"The action of Yang (+) and Yin (-) creates this other force. Yang, which is a male force always thrusting ahead, acts upon Yin, a female force that seeks to contain. At their conjunction the irresistible force meets the immovable object. The pressure of the meeting creates a 3rd force. An example is flint and steel used in fire making. Striking the flint (Yin) with the steel (Yang) causes a spark of energy. All three: Yin, Yang and spark, taken together form the Tao—the world we live in. The world of phenomena—sickness and health.

"The acupuncturist learns to harness this principle for the treatment of disease. He applies this idea to the energies flowing in the human body, which have been mapped by practitioners of Chinese medicine over thousands of years. By applying this Law of Energy and several other principles, the physician is able to treat disease—and help the patient to maintain health.

"Dr. Ju always said that the true healer has to function on three levels. Only by understanding the laws can he treat correctly. He must uderstand:

1. *The underlying cause of disease*
2. *The current disease process*
3. *And he must limit future negative ramifications*—all at the same time.

"It makes perfect sense, if we view a disease pattern as a triangle—we must repair the energy of all three legs at once, since they're obviously connected."

"Energy can't be seen or heard with a stethoscope," I said, "so how can you read my energy just by feeling my wrist?"

The Doc nodded judiciously. It was starting to rain.

I motioned for the girls, then I went on, "When I take my symptoms to a regular doctor and he says, 'Here, take these pills', it makes me nervous. I'm never sure that he knows what's wrong. I don't want to eat strong pills with a lot of side effects—not unless I'm half dead, then I might eat them. But when I see you, and you feel my wrist pulses, I always feel confident that you've really found out what is wrong with me. Then you fix it."

"You're basically pretty healthy," he said.

"Maybe I'm just responsive to this kind of medicine."

Looking disappointed at the rain, Dr. Rosenblatt put on his jacket and picked up the tackle box. No sense getting soaked just because we forgot to listen to the weather report. A large fish splashed into a school of anchovies straight out from where we were standing. "See, there are fish out there today," he observed.

"No doubt about it," I agreed. "It's a big ocean, full of currents."

*

Dr. Ju's Journal—3—Spring, 1969

Now I know how difficult it was for my teachers. Ha, ha. The grand pain for which there is no cure—taking on students. But nobody could be more enthusiastic than my UCLA boys.

Today I taught them the magic of casting the needle. The needle crosses an eternity of space, and then enters the precisely correct acupuncture point—because the healer's energy wills it to. Not because the doctor has only mental knowledge of the points—no, it is a question of chi, of life force.

I showed them how to move the energy with their needle hand, to manipulate the air; but naturally, I didn't give them the needle. Maybe I never will—certainly not until they get the casting technique correct. No sense rushing the mountain.

It is amusing to walk with them in Chinatown on the way to lunch. They practice casting as they walk—so enthusiastic and American; but so nuts. Nobody can do casting while walking. Casting the needle is casting—walking to lunch is walking. At least, they eat dim sum with great enthusiasm, which is good.

And they got the haircut! In a brilliant insight, I said to the Chairman, "When you do the doctor, you must look the doctor." And the Chairman perceived my wisdom. I saw him understand, exactly like I had casted a needle of perception with total accuracy. It pierced his consciousness, which is not a bit slow. And today, no more unsightly hair. Of course, who cares about hair, really? My honored grandfather wore a thick braid down to his buttocks.

*

"There are six pulses in each wrist, and each one represents an organ" the Doc said. We were sitting in his car in the parking lot, watching it rain. "Each wrist holds three pulse positions, with a surface pulse and a deep pulse at each location. Each position relates to an internal organ. Placing my finger tips on the wrist, I move over all the pulses until I complete my picture of the relative strength beating from each organ.

"The pulses are a way of getting me into sync with the patient—physically and almost psychically. It's like I'm touching each organ through my finger tips." Dr. Rosenblatt placed his finger on my right wrist as he'd done many times in the office, but never before at the pier. "Is it hot or cold? How about your intestine," he said pressing with his index finger. "Yours is almost always hot because of all the coffee you drink.

"This is almost like dowsing for information," he laughed. "Each of the twelve pulses tells its own story. When I take them together, they give me the total picture of a person's health."

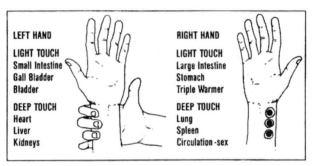

12 Pulse Chart

"The Chinese describe the pulses as sensations in the wrist being transmitted to the physician's fingers like the tension on a bowstring. There's a classic story attributed to Emperor Ling Fu the Wise. The Emperor was kind of a strange guy. Like most patients, he wanted to test his doctor, but the Emperor had divine authority, so he could do all the testing he wanted to. He summoned his physician, Wang Chow, who had a wonderful reputation as a diagnostician.

"I have devised the ultimate test for you," the Emperor said, with an inscrutable smile. "I shall tie a string around my wrist and pass the end through this jeweled ornamental screen. You will stand behind the screen and diagnose by feeling the string. Are you accomplished enough to do that…?"

"Of course, I can do it," Wang Chow answered, without hesitation. He turned on his cotton-soled slippers and walked behind the screen. "Pass me the string, your Holiness," he said.

Emperor Ling Fu the Wise tied the string around the leg of a cow, then passed the loose end through the screen to the physician.

Wang Chow felt the pulse coming down the taut string and after a suitable period of time had elapsed, he announced, "All you need is to eat lots of fresh grass, your Excellency."

Dr. R. chuckled good-naturedly. He liked that story.

"So Wang Chow got more famous and received a big reward...?" I asked.

"Something like that. Diagnosing is a very subtle art. Pulses are extremely subtle. Sometimes they're so weak and thin that you can barely feel them, and sometimes they're like a freight train.

"Which brings us to another interesting point," he said. "The Concept of Relative Strength. A germ, or a disease, will always seek out the weakest organ to attack. We call it Affinity of Vibrations."

"You mean a germ has a vibration, and it seeks out the organ with the same vibration to attack?" I chuckled at the absurdity.

"Very much so," he answered, seriously. "Everything has a vibration rate. Normally your stomach, for instance, has a healthy vibration. But you go to a dance party. Due to a heavy intake of alcohol and sugar, your stomach is weakened and now its vibration rate has fallen dramatically. Germs are everywhere, of course. Let's say one of the musicians, the sax player, has a dose of flu germs. If your immune had maintained its normal strong vibration, the wayward germs would have bounced off; but rum and coke weakened your stomach. The flu germs found a nice little home at the lower vibration and moved right in."

"And you can feel this weakened state through the pulses in a patient's wrist?" I asked.

"Right, the pulses and the sparkle in their eye. If a person becomes sensitive to the energy level of her body, and comes in for treatment when she feels out of balance, then she probably won't get sick. There's a Chinese proverb that translates something like: "Only the inferior physician must treat the disease he was not proficient enough to prevent." The Doc grinned charmingly, and tipped his head back to survey the sheets of rain pounding on the window. The girls were in the back seat, playing some kind of girl game. All was well, and we were on our way to lunch.

*

Dr. Ju's Journal—4—Autumn, 1969

A doctor is always conventional—part of the community—not some kind of odd-ball. For instance, I want to buy a pair of cowboy boots. It would make me feel almost ecstatic to swagger down the street like John Wayne, but it is not possible. I am a Chinese doctor, not a cowboy. Image is very important.

Chapter One

The winds of politics and style must blow past the doctor without ruffling his chin whiskers.

Today, as the winter rains come calling, the omens are totally right at last. Rain was on the window when I looked out and saw Kathy, the Chairman's wife, with the three boys. That was the vision-dream. All four of them standing on the little porch in the rain. Now, we can begin.

Of course, they are not married yet. It is almost unbearably mysterious how these things work. I had my vision fourteen years ago in Canton Province and only now is it coming true. So very unworldly. Here I am, a normal man—interested in many things, but basically very normal—ask anybody. And here they are, four students from a different culture with very different ways—and here we are locked together because of a vision from the future. Locked together, almost like I am their father, teaching them the ways of medicine and good health. Very, very strange.

But it's quite unlucky that she is named Kathy. I can not say that "th" sound no matter how hard I practice. Nobody of culture can say it. I try, I try; but all I can make my mouth say is Kaffy. They smile. And Bill, with two ridiculous "Ls" on the end. It's embarrassing, for no good reason. Why can't they have normal names? I hate being smiled at. Kaffy and Birr. Why don't they have a sensible name like Bao or Ming?

I made it a little difficult for them to learn from me. I suggested that they had to raise a sizable amount of money for the teacher before we could begin formal classes—and they each have to bring one more student. Ah, these little tests—where would real teachings be without them?

And can you believe it? They cleverly raised more money than I had asked for by using the tools at their disposal. Kathy made a flyer with a flaming Buddha on it and they plastered it all over

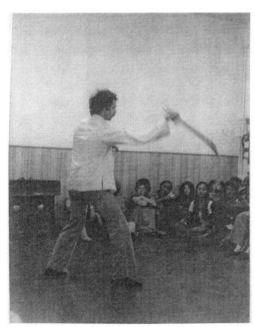

Steven demo with Broad Knife

the UCLA campus. They drew a sizable crowd to a series of lectures given by Marshall Ho'o and me and another friend from Chinatown, Kai Di, the well known actor, who is also an expert on I Ching. We were their money making tools. It was arranged for each of us to lecture on consecutive weeks at their UCLA in a huge auditorium, where they charged the audience to hear us talk about strange Chinese things. Marshall talked about Chinese cooking. Everyone loved it. Marshall does have good English.

Embarrassingly, I was forced to use a translator. Who knows how accurately my words were relayed? The audience was polite enough to clap. Anyway, the lecture series was a great success. They have the money, several thousand, in a bank account especially for the classes. Now I have to teach the class, which of course I want to. They will rent a lecture room—not as large as UCLA.

Beautiful place, UCLA. First time I ever went there.

* * *

Chapter Two

Energy at Birth

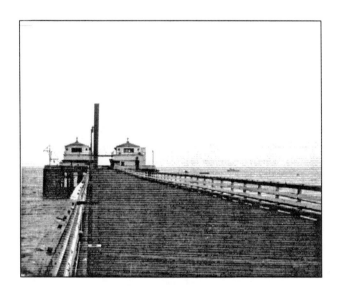

"Where does the energy come from to treat patients?" I asked the Doc.
"Come from…?"
"Do you give energy with the needles, or what?"
"No, not exactly."

Dr. Ju's Journal—5—Late Autumn, 1969

Looking out from the podium, I paused a moment, wondering if they knew? Eight downturned faces, all frantically scribbling notes on the initial lecture

I was giving. Two young women and six men. The future of medicine. Yes, I think they perceive it dimly. Most of them have that tiny glow of cognition.

From tonight onward, each person here will spread the message of health, and in a few years the ripples on this little pond will build into a tidal wave, splashing into all corners of medicine. It's exciting, in a way. A whole, big country ready and eager for change, and only these eight have an inkling. Nine counting myself. And only myself and three of my esteemed teachers knew of my vision. That makes twelve—the Zodiac. And Ancestor Lu, of course, who sent the vision.

It is so easy to lose sight of the magical part of this world. Even if you never miss a day of meditation, the normal, mundane weight of responsibility can overwhelm you. You can actually forget an earth-shakingly important vision for years at a time—just like it never happened. No joke! I, myself, had completely forgotten everything except doing the doctor and raising my family. Very frightening. Humans hang by such a delicate thread. What if Marshall Ho'o hadn't tricked me into attending the demonstration with the lure of finding a few new clients?

To remember that evening of Marshall's demonstration always makes me smile. The Chairman did a routine with the Taoist broad knife, looking like an electrifying barbarian demon with hair and mustache flying—then something about him blasted me out of my torpor. Blasted! Like the top of my head opened up and there was my vision again, fully blown. And three of those T'ai Chi players at that insignificant little demonstration were in my vision. Four, if you count me. Unexplainable! Fantastic!! Utterly mind-blowing, in the jargon of my new students.

So I went over to talk to them.

*

"Each person has his own personal bio-electrical energy field surrounding him," Dr. Rosenblatt continued in answer to my question. "At the moment of conception when a sperm enters the egg, the female and male properties come together (Yin/Yang), and the third force (the Tao, the magical combining energy) results in a baby.

"The baby comes complete with a set of organs and energy channels, similar to the parents, but distinctly its own. At birth, every baby has the strengths and weaknesses that she'll live with the rest of her stay on Earth. And she's filled with energy—flowing with energy that is predictable, and moves along defined channels (the meridians) that can be adjusted to correct imbalances. Every living thing has a life energy grid that keeps the physical body knitted together. This energy pattern *can* be strengthened to prevent disease and to prolong healthy life."

"I think people are put off by the idea of having needles stuck in them," I mentioned, changing the flow of conversation. "Even if they'd like to be cured or strengthened, they're afraid of needles."

"Yes, they are frightened," he said. "That's one reason I've gone on as many TV shows as possible. I try to de-mystify acupuncture. If I show the TV camera that the needles are as fine as a blonde hair, it makes the audience less nervous . If a person is treated once, he knows there's virtually no pain, then the fear goes away. You're not afraid anymore, are you?" he asked.

"No," I testified. "It hurts as much as a love pinch. Some needles don't hurt at all. Sometimes I can't even feel them go in. It depends on where you stick them."

"The shape of the acupuncture needle is the reason," the Doc explained. "A hypodermic needle is cut on a bevel and is hollow; but an acupuncture needle is rounded at the tip and shaped like, well, like a needle. Hypodermic needles actually core the skin tissue as it pierces, and then it injects a liquid which further bothers the tissue. An acupuncture needle is so thin that it pushes the cells aside, slipping between them. That's why the acupuncture needle seldom causes bleeding or bruising, and rarely causes pain. It slips into the skin, unlocking a stuck part of the energy pattern, like a key inserted into a lock."

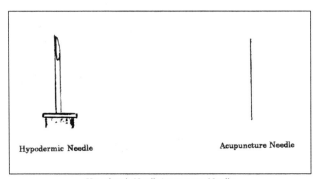

Hypodermic NeedleAcupuncture Needle

"The pattern is what is important. The needle is only a lever. Actually, acupuncture points are like funnels, drawing in energy from the outside. As long as they are open, good health is automatic. But if several funnels get blocked, we have to use some form of treatment to unblock them. Sometimes the unblocking of this energy can produce sudden and seemingly miraculous results.

For instance, the government of Mexico invited me to tour their hospitals from La Paz to Mexico City giving lectures and demonstrations about energetic medicine. When I got to the large Social Security Hospital in Mexico City, the resident doctors picked out their most difficult case, a guy who had been immobilized with back pain for six weeks. They had no idea how to treat him. He couldn't move even an inch without excruciating pain. All he could do was lie there and suffer.

"After I'd given the doctors the required talk on how acupuncture works, they took me up to the chronic pain clinic. Three interns had to lift the fellow up and turn him onto his stomach—the pain didn't allow him to move by himself. I treated him with a series of back points along the bladder meridian that seemed appropriate.

"At the end of about ten minutes of treatment, he started flexing his body. "It feels better," he said, gingerly. The doctors' mouths fell open one after another. He was moving his arms and legs. Then this guy actually sat up!

"Hey, take it easy!" everybody yelled at him.

"Lay back down and I'll treat you a little more," I offered.

"When I finished, he sat up again. Then he stood up before anyone could stop him. "It doesn't hurt!" he yelled. "It doesn't hurt…!" He started running around his bed and jumping up and down!

"Needless to say, the doctors and nurses were flabbergasted. This was a real tough case that they'd thrown at the gringo. They went bonkers with excitement like the cure was a miracle. Un milagro..!"

The Doc chuckled.

"I've had quite a few of these "miracle cures," he said, still chuckling to himself. "People are always hobbling in on a cane, then throwing it away after a couple of treatments. The funny part is, that's what I expect to happen. I assume they're all going to get well as the energy is rebalanced. When somebody doesn't respond, that's much more unusual.

The doctor was warming up on this "miracle" business. He had a sort of far away look on his face, like he was remembering pleasant memories.

"My *first* miracle was pretty wild," he said. "It was back in 1971, when I was still studying with Dr. Ju. A middle-aged Anglo fellow wearing work clothes walked into his office at the back of the Chinatown apartment, very respectfully, with his hat in his hand. He said his ten year old son had been riding a bicycle when a car hit him. The boy was now in the hospital in a coma. He wanted Dr. Ju to go cure him.

"Understand that Dr. Ju wanted nothing to do with hospitals, since he didn't have a license of any kind. There were no acupuncture licenses. Officially, this form of medicine didn't exist. He pointed at me and introduced me to the man. "This is my #1 Assistant," he said, confidently. "He will take care of the boy."

"Well, I didn't have a license either. Nobody did. In any case, I wanted to help, so I drove over to the hospital during evening visiting hours. Naturally, I was full of trepidation as the father snuck me into the back door of the hospital. You can't work at a hospital without a license. They could put you in jail. But anyway, we rode up the service elevator with my little case of needles in my coat pocket. The kid was in bed, in a coma, unconscious. The hospital staff had no idea in the world how to help him. He'd been there over a month, and was making no progress.

"The father stood guard. "Nobody's coming in this door until you're done," he said steadfastly. He stretched his arms out across the closed doorway. "I'm going to make sure of it." He was serious. It was touching and brave. He stood there like a rock.

Feeling safe from interruption, I treated his son with a needle at the crown of his head, one at the depression on the upper lip and several needles at the alarm points on the fingers of both hands. Right away the boy started moving his arms and legs, which showed he was coming around. The father was ecstatic, and actually, so was I!

"We snuck in to treat him three or four more times, and after that the boy was well enough to go home. Since they didn't know I'd been treating him, the doctors really did think that one was a miracle. The father couldn't thank me enough—brought us home-grown fruit for years. Bushels of it. The boy didn't recall even being in the hospital. He remembered waking up at home. I treated the family for other disorders as time went by. I got to know them really well."

This was great stuff, I decided, jotting madly in my notebook.

"Another funny story," Dr. Rosenblatt related, "was a sweet older gentleman who came in to be treated for deafness. The man had a constant smile on his face, angelic almost, like you see in the Old Master paintings. However, in order to make him hear, even a little, we had to yell pretty loudly. Old age does weaken the body, but age ailments often are quite repairable. He had a form a sensory-neural hearing loss—which is a weakness of the auditory nerve that runs from the ear to the brain. I used a standard acupuncture treatment that has been developed over the centuries—tonifying the kidneys and treating points around the rim of the ear. In Chinese medical theory the ears are the "windows of the kidneys." Just like the eyes are the "windows of the liver." But more about that later. Back to our patient. When we were finished, he could hear better right away. He kind of skipped around the office smiling and happy. The secretary and I waved good-bye to him, and I assumed everything was fine. But a minute later, he came running back into the office, white as a ghost.

"A bomb..!" he gulped. "Somebody put a bomb in my car..!!"

"We all laughed at him… Couldn't help it. He was really comical!" The Doc was chuckling again, but I didn't get the joke.

"What was funny…?" I asked.

"There was no bomb, of course. I went downstairs with him to check out the bomb, and it was just the normal noise of his engine starting up. The muffler was a little worn, but not even too bad. He could hear it. That was the difference..! It scared the daylights out of him..!"

I found myself empathizing with the old guy. Cars are frightening in the best of times. Maybe he had enemies, real or imagined, who would love to put a bomb in his car. And maybe I should have my ears checked. I often make people repeat what they say to me.

*

Dr. Ju's Journal—6—Winter, 1970

After the class we eat. Talking is hungry making. So is note taking, evidently. We eat with deep relishment to replenish ourselves. The food of the Middle Kingdom is nourishing. And Oolong tea, of course, is perfect for breaking down the grease.

"Pour it in your eating bowl," I suggest. "See how the grease breaks down into tiny round globules. That's the tea. Coffee doesn't do that."

They all stare into their bowls, especially the one called Louie. I like him, he's a strange, humorous guy. Except he insists to use ketchup on his dim sum. That is pretty weird, even for a barbarian. Almost an insult.

"Drink it," I encourage. And they drink their tea.

It is a fine thing for a man in his middle years to have students hanging on his every word. And a responsibility, of course. I should probably learn English somewhat more fluently. There is no reason for them to be forced to hang on my words quite so diligently.

Energy. Everything is energy. This is what they don't know. And what I must explain carefully, so that they understand. Healing energy guides the needle perfectly. Without it, the needle is nothing. It is difficult to believe that—especially here in the West, where tools and the intellect are thought to be everything. But it is true nevertheless. Perfect health comes from perfectly balanced energy—and all the good nutrients.

*

"Don't you have any miracle cure stories for arthritis," I asked Dr. R. "Everybody is always complaining how much they suffer and nothing can help them."

He thought for a few moments. "We do pretty well with osteo-arthritis," he said. "This tough old carpenter came in a few months ago, a salty kind of guy, and he was shot full of arthritis. His upper back, arms, and both shoulders were joint-bound—stiff and painful, and his hands were gnarled. Right away he started complaining that he only came to see me because his girlfriend made him. He assured me that I couldn't possibly do anything helpful. What he had was just old age, and it was a big waste of his valuable time to be here.

"The Chinese feel that one of the main reasons we have so much arthritis," Dr. Rosenblatt explained, "is because we drink so many cold beverages. And we also have a poor diet, with too many milk products.

"Cold slows the energy down. It gets sluggish out in the knuckle joints of the fingers and toes—which is where most arthritis starts. Cold, and also milk fats and calcium causes arthritis to start, they say. The Chinese diet has no dairy and very few iced foods or drinks. Statistically they have far fewer cases of arthritis.

"I wanted to warm the flow of energy to the old carpenter's joint-bound areas, so I lighted a moxa stick. Moxa is a herb called mugwort (artemesia vulgaris) which makes a red ember that burns with a very even heat. I used it to heat up four needles after I inserted them in his shoulders and back to encourage energy to flow across the inflammation blockage in his joints. The inflammation originally started because the knuckles kept getting cold, or so the theory states—then calcium was attracted to the inflammation, which made the knuckles worse. Our body responds to bone inflammation by laying down a layer of calcium to make the bone stronger, which works well on most bones, but not in the joints.

"Personally, I believe that arthritis is mostly energy dysfunction. Stagnant energy causes eddy currents at the finger joints, which allows the normal calcium in the blood to precipitate into the joint. Stagnant energy doesn't flow well over the bump of a joint. Dr. Ju would always rub his hand over the joints in his other hand, and he rubbed his patients' hands, to even out the energy flow over their knuckles.

"Wherever energy doesn't flow evenly, there is pathology (disease). A blockage in an exterior flow of energy is the earliest form of pathology. If the energy is not smoothed out, sooner or later, the function of the connected organ will be disturbed. Then, if the energy flow is not unblocked, there will be damage to the organ itself.

"After four treatments the carpenter was singing my praises. "I've only got a little touch of pain in my upper arm…!" he reported happily. "I can't believe you fixed this. It just kept getting worse for the last fifteen years..!" He was all smiles. So, of course, I was happy, too. Curing people makes quite a good feeling. "Makes happy face," as Dr. Ju used to say.

"But that's osteo-arthritis," the Doc reminded me. "Rheumatoid is very difficult to cure completely."

"Is it connected with rheumatic fever?" I asked.

"No," he said, like perhaps I was an imbecile.

*

Dr. Ju's Journal—7—Winter, 1970

I come from Southern China, from Canton, and because of this I learned many things that students who study only in Beijing probably don't know. I guess you could call it South China folk medicine. Like the Ah Shi *points— which means points on the body that hurt or are sensitive. When somebody touches them, you yell out, "Ah Shi!!" There is a tradition in South China of wise women curers who use one needle to needle the ah shi point that is hurting. It is an effective technique. Thousands of peasants are cured by these women. I knew many of these old healer women in the villages, and learned several good techniques from them. Because I did trading for the monastery in exchange for my medical lessons, I traveled to many villages and whenever I met one of these wise women, I would try to learn what she knew.*

For example, I learned Gwa Sah *from one of these women. Gwa Sah is a method of raising the old blood to the surface of a twisted muscle, so that new, healing, blood can flow in. Gwa Sah is a most useful treatment. Acupuncturists who study the northern methods don't understand this technique very well, but I am going to show my Lo-fan students, so it can become part of their healing skills.*

What exactly is this word, Lo-fan, that I keep talking about? I suppose I should explain it so future historians don't regard me as a total racist. Lo-fan means something like barbarian dog; *but when you are a visitor in the land of the barbarian "Lo-fan" is almost like a term of endearment. It might be translated as "friendly, funny barbarian dog, full of surprises—but don't exactly turn your back on him." That means Lo-fan.*

We Chinese, of course, are among the world's most racist people. We distrust everyone. No one is good enough to marry into our family—not even another Chinese.

*

"Asthma," I said, naming the next topic .

"Puberty," the Doc replied.

"You don't treat puberty," I answered, brilliantly. "It's not an illness."

"Maybe not to you," he said, laughing. "But, the best time to treat asthma is at puberty, especially in girls. Puberty is best because a teenager's energy system is still somewhat unformed—at least environmental factors haven't damaged it completely.

"Asthma symptoms actually respond very well to acupuncture treatment. The main problem is that asthma sufferers often come to the office heavily sedated. That's not so good, because in that state, if I even look at them wrong, they go into an attack. I generally treat them with baby needles, which aren't frightening at all."

"Baby needles?" I asked.

"Yes, very tiny needles that we treat babies with."

"Oh."

"I think my favorite "miracle cure" was that girl in Steamboat Springs," the Doc reflected, with no transition from asthma. "Did I ever tell you about her?"

"I don't know. Was she an asthmatic?"

"She was paralyzed. The girl's father called at the UCLA Acupuncture Clinic soon after we started it and asked if I could go to Colorado to "save his daughter," as he put it. She'd been in a skiing accident and was paralyzed from the waist down with an undiagnosed paralysis. The doctors at the small hospital in Steamboat Springs were afraid to transport her to a large hospital, because nobody was sure what had been damaged.

"One doctor thought it was MS. Another thought it was a herniated disk that might compromise the spinal cord, if she was moved. Nothing was broken. Nothing showed on the X-ray; but of course, that was in the days before CAT scans and MRIs were widely available.

"It was snowing like mad in Colorado and I wasn't wonderfully keen on leaving sunny California. We'd already made a lot of plans for the holidays. But the guy pleaded with me, "Save my daughter, please..! She's been there eight weeks with no cure in sight. The staff seems to love her and care about her, but they aren't helping her!" So I agreed to go. I took Kathleen with me to assist. She likes to ski. That's one thing snow is good for.

"The next morning, we flew to Denver, then changed planes onto a feeble, twin engine local hop that strained up over the Continental Divide. I don't like flying anyway. I'm a nervous flyer. If we were meant to fly, we'd be born with landing gear or something. So I wasn't too overjoyed when the pilot's voice came on, saying we were flying in a non-pressurized cabin. Just then, all the oxygen masks dropped from the ceiling and we sucked oxygen the whole way over the Rocky Mountains. We had a very bumpy ride, but we made it."

"You're still here to tell the tale," I observed, wittily.

"Right. So we landed and checked into a motel, then took a taxi straight to the hospital. The young woman's doctor was very concerned. He confirmed that she'd been there two months already, and he didn't know what was wrong with her. He showed me the X-rays. They revealed nothing abnormal, at all.

"We went in to see the patient. She was sitting in a wheelchair, about twenty years old with long dark hair, cute as could be. And she couldn't move her legs. Not a twitch. No feeling, no movement.

"I listened to the six pulses in each wrist, and what I sensed was a Wood problem (liver, gall bladder) that had resulted in a Kidney Yin deficiency. To confirm my diagnosis, I asked about her menstrual cycle, and she answered that she hadn't had a period for several months. She acted quite surprised that I would ask about her period; but that's what her subtle pulses had told me.

"After quickly planning out a strategy, Kathleen and I began to treat her. It was a very involved treatment using several different yin meridians: kidney, spleen and liver—and the corresponding yang meridians: bladder, stomach and gall bladder. We used electrical stimulation, low-volt electrodes attached to the needles, and Kathleen held burning moxa sticks on the needles to give an extra boost to the energy flow.

"The next morning, we went back to the hospital. The girl was sitting in a wheelchair beside the elevators, waiting for us to arrive. Grinning mysteriously, she wheeled across the marble lobby to meet us.

"Hey, Doctor Rosenblatt, watch this...!" she yelled, standing up and taking eight or ten steps toward us. "I can walk again!"

Two of her nurses grabbed her immediately, one on either side. I thought the nurses were going to faint on the spot. The whole lobby staff started chirping like a flock of excited birds, "Oh, my gosh, she's walking!!" They liked her a lot, and after eight weeks of caring for her, they regarded her almost like family. And it was lucky that the nurses were alert. The girl's leg muscles were quite weak from sitting so long and she probably would have fallen without assistance. She just wanted to show me she could walk, so she came out to demonstrate without telling anyone or asking permission. Nice.

"Anyway, we treated her for a few more days, then she flew home to New Jersey. Kathy even got to spend a few hours on the ski slopes."

"New Jersey?" I asked. "How did her father find you?"

"I don't know. He heard about me somewhere, and tracked me down. A few days after we got home, the father called to thank me. He said his daughter arrived home in time for Passover. It made the family very happy."

"Pretty good story," I allowed.

"That's one of my favorites miracles," the Doc said with a very nice smile.

*

Dr. Ju's Journal—8—Spring, 1970

Kai Ying Tung arrived last week, and he really is a marvel at T'ai Chi Ch'uan. Watching him is like seeing poetry in motion, especially with the swords. His whole family is so important to T'ai Chi that they are almost like princes in China. Grandfather Tung brought Yang Style T'ai Chi from the south to Beijing after the last Yang died.

I took the liberty of inviting young Master Tung over to meet my students. Well, perhaps I tempted him too much with a ready-made class, but he hadn't been in my modest apartment more than ten minutes when he had everybody up and doing T'ai Chi. Pretty bold. I like that. He does the T'ai Chi like I do the doctor. Breathe it. Eat it.

The UCLA boys think Tung is marvelous. I can tell. They're eating it up. They are a strange lot. Mainly they're not Chinese. I shouldn't hold that against them; but it's like they force the teaching to go a certain way, or else they don't want it.

For instance, I suggested to Howard Lee, one of my senior students in the ways of energy, who is also a very accomplished martial artist, that maybe he would please teach my new students a few moves in case somebody bothers them. As if he is their elder brother, teaching them a bit of serious self-defense. I plan to take them around the country with me to do the doctor, and I don't want to worry about their safety. That's pretty simple to understand, isn't it?

But they don't want to. They laugh and won't take it seriously. So Howard Lee loses face, which makes me lose face. We don't care, Howard and me. When you're trying to teach Lo-fan, you're going to lose some face. They just don't know enough to be sensitive. It can't be helped. They laughed because they say we are now in the Age of Peace and Love. Ha, ha. They're learning T'ai Chi so they can be graceful and healthy. Fighting is secondary. Well, maybe they know something. After all, it is their country. "Make love, not war." That is one of their Beatle slogans. It's difficult to argue against making love.

* * *

Chapter Three

Energetics

"What are Energetics?" Dr. Rosenblatt asked, and then answered the question. "Energetics are the rules that energy follows. One might say that everything Dr. Ju tried to teach us related to Energetics as they apply to health and disease in the body.

"In a way, Energetics is our mind's attempt to put some structure on the vast and swirling ocean of energy that exists in each of us, so that we can hope to control some part of it.

"This particular attempt at a structure has taken place over centuries in China. Dr. Ju was heir to eons of practical experimenting on energy. He succeeded in passing some of this knowledge on to us.

"If works, keep—if no good, throw out!" This was one of Dr. Ju's favorite sayings referring to medical theory. We heard it over and over, and this saying defines the core approach of Chinese medicine—a relentless trial and error leading to a very practical body of medical arts.

"The Chinese make a theory as a spotlight to locate interesting phenomena—and then work with the observation to see how it can be applied. In Western Medicine, we see several phenomena, then we piece them together to come up with a theory about what we saw. These are two completely different approaches to science.

"For instance, the Chinese rarely did any dissecting. Instead, they would come up with a theory of functional relationship (how things work together) and then run innumerable experiments over generations to prove or disprove the theory."

"Do you mean that within the Taoist monasteries medical experimenting was orderly for many, many generations in spite of wars, famines and floods?" I asked.

"Absolutely. They had an unbroken lineage of perhaps two thousand years, or maybe more. And some monasteries are still functioning. In 1973, Dr. Ju took Kathleen and me to visit a monastery outside of Hong Kong that was definitely still functioning as a warehouse for information. That monastery is at least a thousand years old. In a thousand years, there is time for quite a few experiments.

"Here's what I mean by a functional relationship. Long ago, a Chinese doctor noticed that the lungs must absorb something from the air by breathing, and then expel used air. The intestine also absorbs body fuel from food, and passes on the waste products. The lung and the large intestine are both fed by what flows down the esophagus and the trachea (wind pipe and the food pipe). The Chinese then proposed a theory that the lungs and large intestine are connected. Western medicine would not usually look in this direction; but as an acupuncturist, I see that patients who have an intestinal problem often have an upper respiratory problem as well. I see this over and over, and to me this clearly makes a good case for the theory."

"Wow," I said.

"Those old Chinese doctors observed themselves and their patients—then they started putting tidbits of observed information together to expand and verify a theory. They saw that people with intestinal problems often have breathing problems—and if that wasn't bad enough, they also found that both of those illnesses seem connected to skin rashes.

"Oddly, we find today that intestinal problems are also the source for sinus problems. And what are the sinuses? The first part of the respiratory system. In fact, the Chinese say that allergy problems (both skin and sinus) begin in the gut. They call this a functional cluster. Both systems control the same kinds of tissue. (The lining of the lungs, and the lining of the intestine are very similar tissues—mucus membranes, thin tissue meant for absorption.)

"During the time when The National Acupuncture Association ran the Acupuncture Clinic at UCLA, we did a study on the effect of acupuncture on childhood asthma. We were working directly with the Director of Pediatric Pulmonary Medicine. My job was to analyze the medical charts of the children we were considering for the study to see if there were any reasons to exclude any of the kids. If they were hemophiliacs—we weren't going to stick needles in them, for instance.

"I noticed that a tremendous number of the kids with asthma had intestinal problem (40% of them) such as ulcerative colitis, Crohne's disease, irritable bowel syndrome, which is a much higher percentage than you would find in a normal population. *Or* they had chronic skin problems (psoriasis, eczema) which are severe itching rashes.

"I took these observations to the professor and asked, "Have you noticed the high incidence of intestinal problems in this grouping of asthmatics? And they also have skin problems."

""Poppycock," he answered. "It's just pure chance.""

*

"From these functional relationships, the Chinese derived the Laws of Energetics. These laws express the relationship between the various organ systems and their energy flows.

"Each organ system not only consists of the physical organ (Large Intestine) but it also includes the meridian—which is the energy surrounding and flowing through the organ. In other words, the energy flowing along the meridian animates the organ, which becomes a dynamic center for *that* energy. For instance, the heart is very full of heart energy.

"If one has an operation to remove a damaged organ, like the gall bladder, the energy of the meridian still flows, but no longer has a physical organ to reflect in, and so therefore is much weakened."

Dr. Ju's Journal—10—Spring, 1970

To do the doctor, you must have a large gall bladder. In Chinese medicine, the gall bladder is responsible for courage and leadership—the leader is someone who can *absorb everyone's insecurities and anxieties, and still gather the forces together to forge a direction.*

This is a key teaching in doing the doctor. I tell them frequently; but they look blank at me. You have to focus on the patient to be attuned to the anxieties that surround the illness—and show them a way out of the maze. This is a big feature.

Gall bladder is courage—forging forward. Gall bladder is yang. One of the ridiculous things about Western medicine is if gall bladder get a problem—take out and throw away. That is ridiculous! That is not medicine!! I teach my students to fix the problem, not cut out and throw away.

*

"Yin-Yang is the fundamental principle of inside and outside, hollow (yang) and solid (yin) forms the major energetic functional relationship between the 12 organ systems."

"But how do things work together, really?" I asked. "How can I see the relationship of Yin and Yang in myself?"

"Well," the Doc said, pursing his lips. "That is deeply sought after knowledge. But consistent with functional Chinese medical theory, the Yang meridians run from Heaven down to Earth—that is from the head down the body to the feet, while the Yin meridians run upward toward Heaven—from the feet up the body to the head.

"In Chinese medical texts, man is pictured standing on the Earth with his hands stretched above his head toward Heaven. This illustrates the three Upper Yin meridians, which begin in the breast and rise up through the fingers toward Heaven.

"The Lung Meridian (Yin) begins in the chest and rises to the thumb, as it it stretched high above the head. Its coupled Yang (Large Intestine) begins on the index finger and descends from this Heavenly position down to the Intestines.

"The Upper Yins start in the breast and the Upper Yangs start in the fingers, and run into the face, with internal connections that run into the organs themselves."

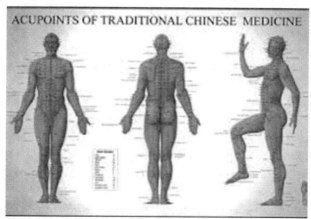

Diagram of Meridians See end of chapter for individual meridian diagrams.

"The Liver Meridian (Yin, one of three) start at the foot and comes up into the chest area—and the upper Yin (Lung, for instance) takes off and runs to the fingers. These pairings work in a sequence of Lower Yins, feeding the Upper Yin. The energy changes at the apex and becomes Yang, which then descends to the face and then descends again to the foot. All the Yang meridians begin or end on the face—All Yin meridians begin or end on the chest—depending on whether they are upper or lower.

"The face is the middle junction point between the upper and lower Yangs. The Chest is the middle junction for the upper and lower Yins.

All the meridians begin or end on the toes or fingers. It's as if we are woven on a loom. The warp and whoof threads hold us together."

"Woven," I said, finally getting it. "Is this what the figure eight diagram you keep drawing is about?" Over the years, the Doc has attempted to explain this concept to me probably more than twenty times. I have versions of this vaguely man-shaped figure 8 all through my notes. Now, the nickel had dropped. It's like a weaver's shuttle trailing a line of energy (the woof) being thrown back and forth over the stationary warp threads, thus making the woven fabric—making the energy pattern for the flesh of the body to grow on.

"Well, yes," he answered, drawing another eight-shaped diagram. "The lower Yin meridians begin on the toes and end on the chest, where the upper Yin meridians take over and reach to the fingers. Earth energy becoming Heaven bound equals Yin. Yang equals Heavenly energy seeking the Earth.

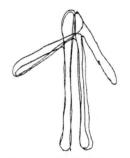

Energetic Body Pattern

"Practically speaking, Yang is hot and Yin is cold," the Doc said. "You can go out in the coldest weather, and your face is not cold, relatively. That's why clothing is worn on the rest of the body in cold weather, but lastly on the face. The head is the Yang of Yangs, and the hands are the second Yang juncture box, which explains why the hands rarely need to be covered with gloves until the weather becomes very cold.

"The opposite cold receptivity occurs at the Yin junction areas of the chest and feet. Everyone knows that a cold almost always starts when the ankles and feet get cold, or the chest is left open to a cold wind. That's how it is, because Yin is cold, and Yang is hot. Yin and Yang are the warp and woof threads. This explains the meridians and how they flow energetically."

The Doc thought for a moment, organizing his thoughts, I guess. "So far I've been talking only about the twelve major meridians. Let's try to understand the whole energetic map of the body for a minute.

"The freeways of energy are the twelve major flows—then there are city streets, alley ways and even foot paths along the river and through vacant lots.

"Only the twelve major meridians are anchored in organs. That is the reason for their size and importance. Just as there are major arteries ending in capillaries for blood flow—so the enegy system is organized in the exact same tree of life."

*

Dr. Ju's Journal—11—Summer, 1970

Bill is also a funny guy, and smart, too. They still kid him about the cat scratch fever. He takes kidding pretty well. He has a good strong ego—kind of an innate self-worth—that allows him to be kidded and used as a demonstration subject. He likes to think of himself as sensitive, and, of course, he is—which is going to make him a good practitioner. And he's also deathly afraid of needles, which is pretty amusing for an acupuncture student, and he's a hypochondriac as well. Nicely complex. He should be able to recognize patient's suffering. Yes, Prensky and the Chairman are nicely turned out. Both of them have a chance to be whole, completed beings—or close to it. We'll see what fate has in store for them.

But anyway, I like to use Bill for a demonstration dummy. He's very responsive, and doesn't die of mortification. That first class was a beauty. They still don't know what hit them.

Bill's cat had scratched him, quite a few times actually, and the scratches were a little festered and red. Very normal. But Bill was showing his cronies and was getting agitated about the possibility of having cat scratch fever—whatever the heck that is—some new beatnik disease he was worried about. Finally, he got around to showing me. I said I would cure him.

Before he had a chance to get nervous or run away, I needled him in several points on his right arm. All my new students were watching—so attentively—as I slipped needles in perfectly. Putt, putt, putt. Then I returned to organizing my lecture notes from which I had been interrupted.

I looked up a minute later, ready to start the lecture and Bill was gone. "Where you go..?" I remember asking. It had only been a few seconds. He couldn't have walked off with needles in his arm, could he?

Well, I wouldn't put any craziness past these people; but in this case, Bill had not walked off. He had slumped to the floor. His friends were looking at him in a very worried manner.

Truthfully, he did look terrible. Gray and clammy. He had passed out. Men are sometimes overly delicate in their electrical system. I usually like to treat them lying down, but this was hardly a treatment, just a couple of points to pump up his immune system. Women are much stronger electrically. They seldom pass out.

All my new students were poised—waiting for me to do something, so I did. "No worry, I fix," I told them and to fix him, I pulled the needles from his arm and stuck two of them into points on the side of his knee.

Happily, Bill came back to life. Instantly. It was a grand performance. He sat up. His pink color came right back. He blinked his eyes and said, "Let's go." I remember that's what he said. That odd statement. "Let's go." I guess he was ready for the lecture to start. So I started.

Believe me, they were all flabbergasted by that demonstration. I acted like it was completely normal—like perhaps I had knocked him out, then brought him back to life, on purpose. Cheesh, I hate it that males are so delicate. What if he had hurt himself when he fell over? Everything would have been ruined on Day One of the lecture series.

*

The following pages contain 14 diagrams of the major acupuncture lines…

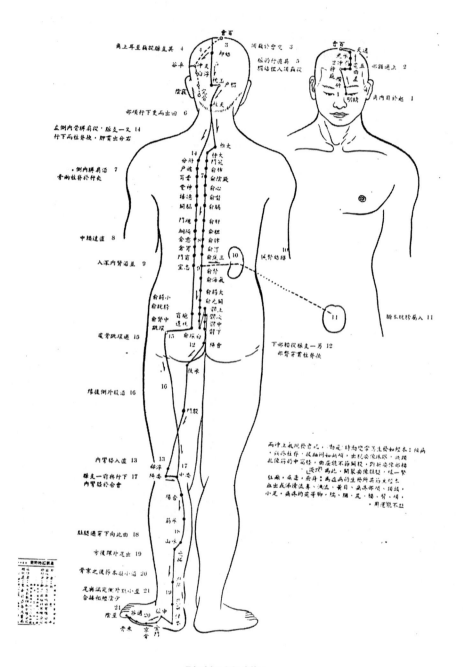

Bladder Meridian

Chapter Three

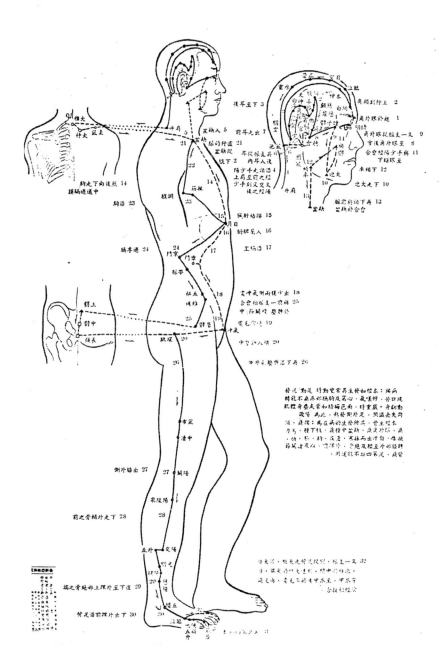

Gallbladder Meridian

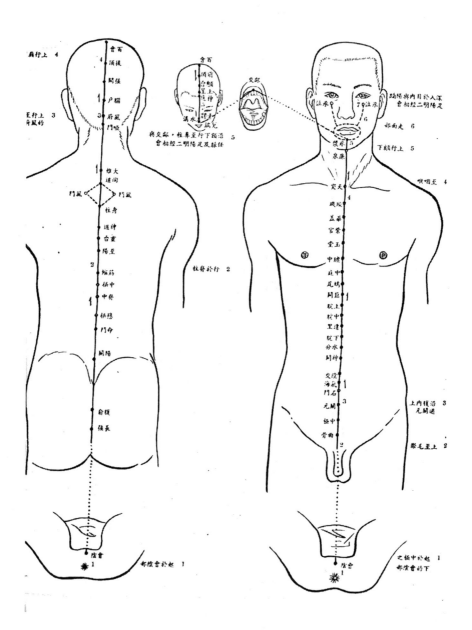

Governing Vessel and Conception Vessel

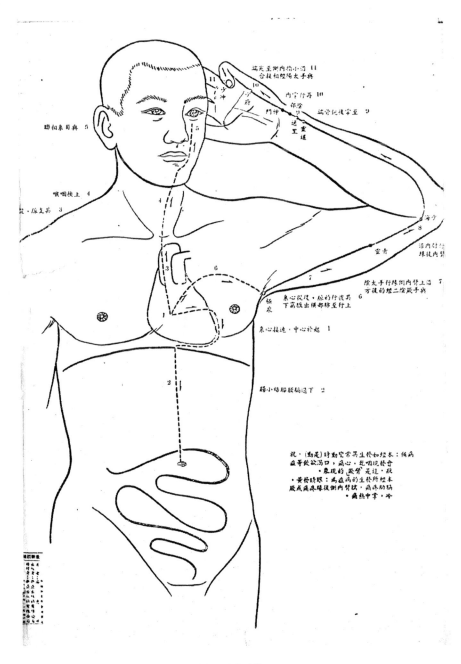

Heart Meridian

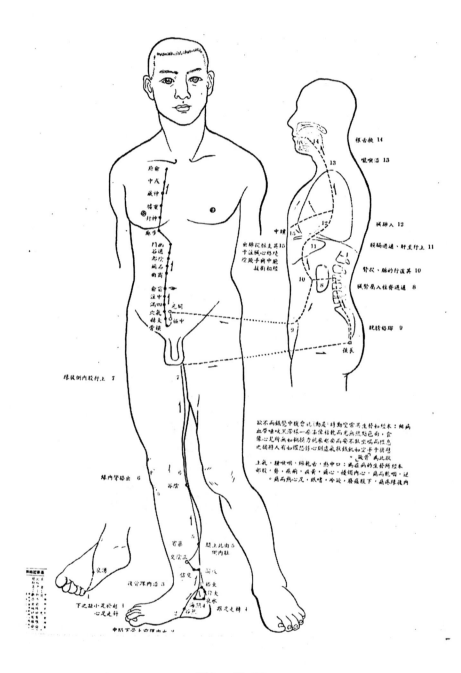

Kidney Meridian

CHAPTER THREE

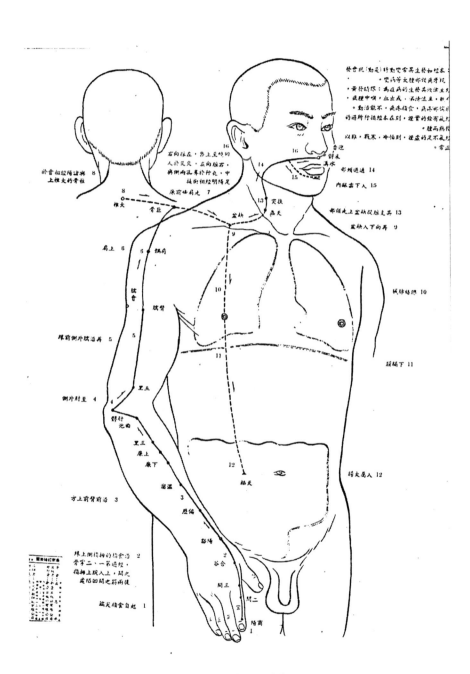

Large Intestine Meridian

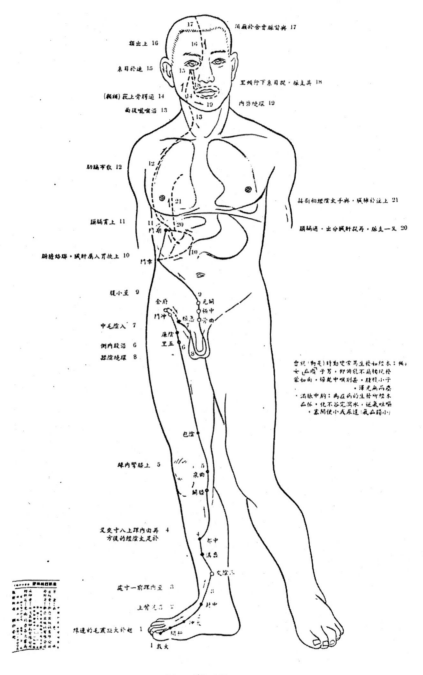

Liver Meridian

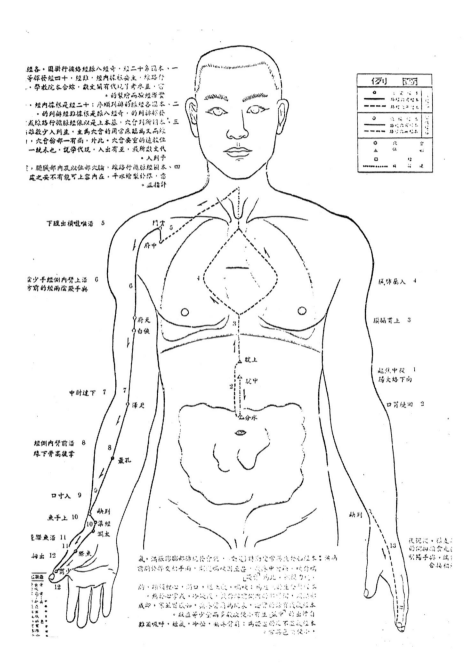

Lung Meridian

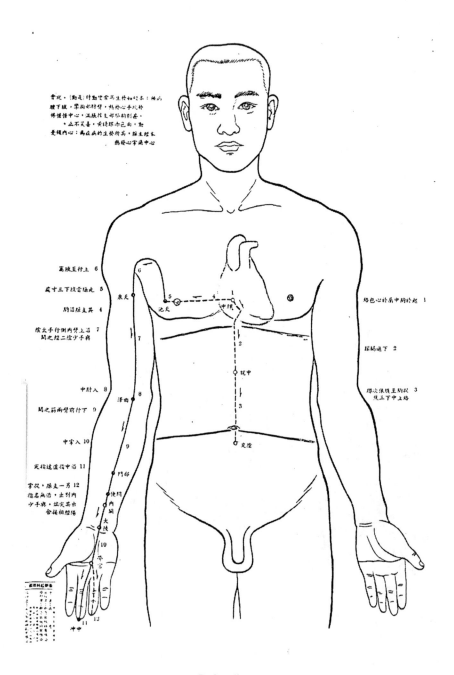

Pericardiam

Chapter Three

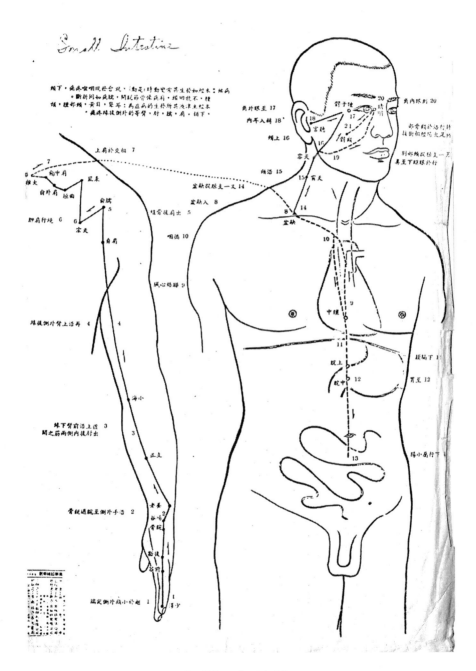

Small Intestine Meridian

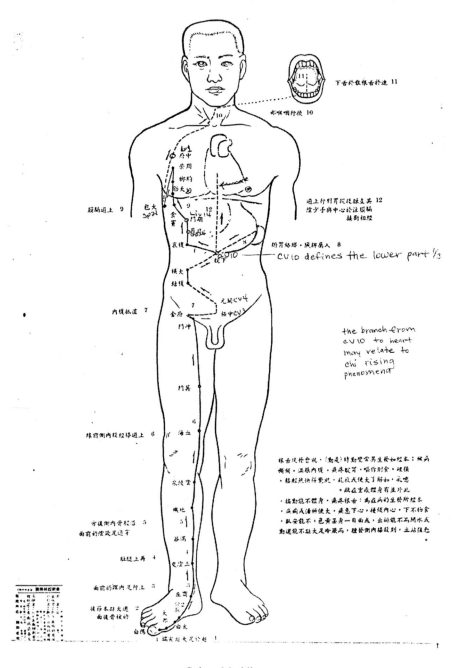

Spleen Meridian

Chapter Three

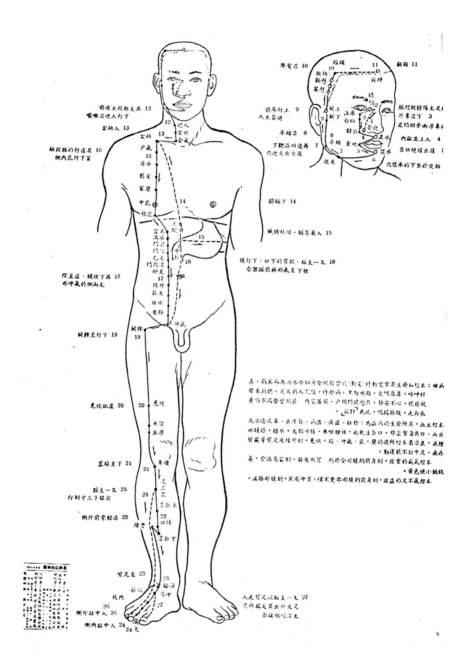

Stomach Meridian

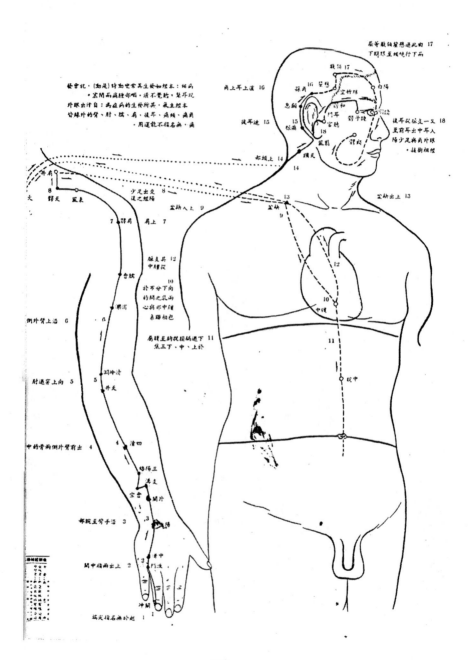

Triheater

Chapter Four

Energetics 2A

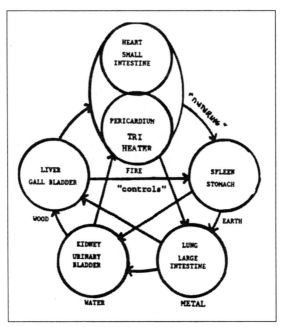

Five Elements chart

Dr. Ju's Journal—12—Spring, 1970

Every day they come over. They watch me treat patients. I show the energy points or something useful. Next week I will begin teaching them Five Elements. I think they are ready to grasp it. After I am done with morning patients, we take the walk and eat dim sum. In some foods they are still a little squeamish, but they are good sports. I like them. They make me laugh.

I like to eat chicken feet several times a week. They are chewy and delicious, and very good for the ligaments and joints. Think about it—chicken feet are mostly bones and ligaments—that's all. So I tell them that eating chicken feet is good for T'ai Chi players because chickens are good fighters, and their feet are the fighting part. It makes sense. So now we get two orders. Everybody gnaws the bones.

We have a small recurring joke. As a teaching parable, I one time said, "If somebody bothers you, you give them chicken feet." Meaning, use the strength and ligament power of chicken feet if you ever get in a scrape, like fighting cocks do. The boys thought that was funny. Now, every time we order chicken feet, one of them will chime up with the saying. Louie likes to say it to the serving girls, who of course don't understand a word of English.

*

Five Elements Theory

"The Chinese describe different phases of energy by using a notation called Five Elements. These elemental phases of energy are:

Fire
Earth
Metal
Water
Wood

"Each of these elements illustrates a certain way that energy acts. Combined they are a theory of Cycles of Energy Movement—each cycles into the other. Each one vitalizes a quality of energy.

Yang Fire is hot flames. Yin fire is expansive, the inside of a bowl. The beating heart is yin fire, contracting, then pushing out.

Yang Earth is deep. Yin Earth is fecund—nourishing, growth.

Yang Metal is sharp. Yin Metal is malleable. It's soft like gold. You can pound it into shapes.

Yang Water is a bubbling brook. Yin Water is a deep dark lake.

Yang Wood is a young green oak. Yin Wood is flowering shrub."

"These energies are usually described in a circle or *creation cycle*, where each energy in turn gives birth to the next phase:

Fire gives birth to Earth. It burns fuel to produce Earth as ashes.

Earth produces Metal. Metals are formed as crystals in the Earth.

Metals oxidize and give birth to Water. (The Chinese had to stretch a bit to get that. But these elementals are analogies to express energetic relationships)

Water gives birth to Wood, the only living element. Basically, this is how the Oriental theories differ from the Medieval Four Elements—the Chinese tend to include life in theories about life.

Finally, Wood gives birth to Fire by combusting, and that completes the circle."

CREATION CYCLE

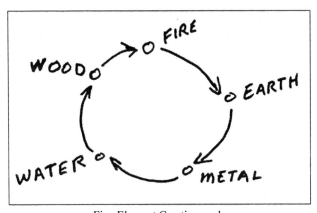

Five Element Creation cycle

"Additionally, the elements across the circle from each other tend to exert a control. For example, Metal controls Wood by cutting it, like an axe would cut a log. Wood controls Earth with its tree roots using nutrients. Earth controls Water by damming its flow. Water controls Fire by quenching, and Fire controls Metal by melting it. It's a naturalistic way of seeing relationships.

"Which coincidentally makes a pentagram, the alchemist's symbol of life. The fact that Wood is a living element has always made this theory come to life for me in a way that early Western medical theories never did.

"They're all metaphors. The large intestine isn't made of metal." he held up a knife from the plate of pumpkin muffins we were eating. "I say it's yang metal, but it's only a way to describe the feeling of the element metal."

Control Points

"Two basic principles of Yin/Yang are Expansion (Yang) and Contraction (Yin). At any one time, an Element Phase gives birth to the Next Phase, and is controlled by the Opposite Phase.

Each element has Yin and Yang aspects to an organ.

Fire Yang is Small Intestine
Fire Yin is Heart
Earth Yang is Stomach
Earth Yin is Spleen
Metal Yang is Large Intestine
Metal Yin is Lungs
Water Yang is Bladder
Water Yin is Kidney
Wood Yang is Gall Bladder
Wood Yin is Liver

"Each meridian as we mentioned in the last chapter has a Yin or Yang aspect. And additionally, *every* meridian has five points that are Elemental Points. For instance, there is a Wood Point on the Fire Meridian, and a Water Point on the Earth Meridian.

Each meridian has Element Points of *all* the Elements. All of these Elemental points are on the *arm below the elbow* and on the *leg below the knee*."

"Recall that I talked about the energy flow slowing down in the fingers and toes—then it turns around for its return journey. By its nature, this slowing and turning energy is very responsive to being manipulated with an acupuncture needle. Needling these Elemental Points causes predictable changes in the flow of energy in most human beings."

Mother/Son Points

"Mother and Son Points are very useful in treating. Using the Mother's Point on a given Son's meridian acts to tonify (or stimulate) that meridian.

"The Rule of Treatment states: *Treat the deficient meridian*. For example, the kidney meridian is weak in many older people. We treat this by pulling the Mother's energy (in this case lung, Metal) into the Son's meridian (Water), thus tonifying the kidney meridian. The needle is placed in the metal point on the water meridian and the kidney energy is strengthened.

"Conversely, using the Son's Point on the Mother's Meridian sedates the Mother. An example of this is stomach upset caused by spicy food or too much tension at the dinner table. The imbalance is calmed by manipulating the Son's Point (Earth Point on the Metal Meridian, near the elbow) and pulling his energy into the Mother's Earth Meridian to treat the stomach.

*

Dr. Ju's Journal—13—Summer, 1970

Very, very interesting, the ebb and the flow. I leave everything to come to America where there is no culture. Here is nice weather, and Hollywood cowboys making money, money, money selling cars and TV sets to immigrants who buy everything so they can be an American. Immigrants who want to buy anything to fill the hole left by this "no culture" no family, no tradition, no monasteries. First Chinese and Japanese, then Korean. Pretty soon they will bring Vietnamese—and probably even the mountain tribes who are being massacred. The melting pot. All come here like a giant magnet pulls them. Why? How can I step back far enough to see the harmony of nature at work? How can anybody?

My students want me to answer these pressing political issues. Because I have yellow skin and Chinese eyes, they think I should know more about Viet Nam than they do. And they really do need the information to plan their future. But how can I know? I am Chinese. The heart of China is Taoist. The heart of Viet Nam is Buddhist. They are not enemies, these two great traditions; but they are not the same.

"I am a doctor," I say, when they ask. "Healing is learnable—is teachable. Politics is a fascinating maze. If he stumbles in, even a genius can't find his way out. Are you a genius?"

That stops them. Ha, ha. These boys all think they're a genius. Maybe so. A young doctor needs a big ego. So maybe they are a genius. But even a genius gets lost in politics.

So I leave everything to come here, and suddenly after a long, dry time, I have everything again. Even rich Anglo sick people are coming to my humble living room. Good students, paying clients. My father has a little house in Fresno. He's slightly happy up there. My children are going to American schools. They are slightly happy. But me…? I am very happy just now. Maybe I'll even buy some cowboy boots.

*

"These meridian relationships provide a fascinating example of how nature has engineered the characteristics of the human energetic system. The Ying and Yang paired meridians go down the body together, interweaving an interlocking energy sequence of Control Aspects where the two lines converge. The Creation Aspects move along the main lines.

"The electrical system is balanced between these two Aspects (Control and Creation) from the yinest of the yin to the yangest of the yang. The dance of energy is held in place by the interlocking aspects as it courses up and down the body."

"I recently treated a woman who had an electrical problem, she was dizzy all the time. She was referred to me by a colleague at Cedars-Sinai Hospital who knew a little acupuncture and realized that it was probably the right treatment, but he didn't know enough himself, so he sent the woman to me. He was right. It was a perfect case.

"She been through every test at Cedars, MRI and CT scans. She had also been to the well-known House Clinic in Los Angeles to have her ears checked. Nothing amiss showed up on any of the tests. The woman was a few years past sixty, and she really staggered on her way to taking a chair in my office.

"Is the room spinning around?" I asked.

"No, the room isn't spinning. I just can't walk straight," she said. "I feel dizzy when I sit up or stand up."

"As we chatted for a few minutes, I realized she had an electrical problem—a good example of a short circuit. There was no disease. No organ was malfunctioning—but she was dizzy, staggering when she walked.

"I did a full Western exam, heart beat, blood pressure, ears, eyes. Nothing showed up; but when I checked her Chinese wrist pulses, I felt a subtle liver imbalance. That was the only indicators that something was wrong, but it was enough to give me the clue on how to proceed. Once I had the clue, the actual treatment was very straight forward, just a few points on the liver and governing vessel meridians.

"The woman came back for another treatment the next week. She reported that by the time she had gotten off the table from the first treatment, she felt herself getting better. After dinner that first night, she said she had recovered 95 percent. She even said that she had tried to make herself dizzy by jumping up and down, and whipping her head around, but she couldn't. She was basically well.

"Good," I said to her.

"Now, I've got this pain in my foot," she said. "What can you do with that?"

This was a rather perfect example of how acupuncture has grown in the last thirty years. A major hospital was able to refer this woman to the best treatment for her problem, and she was open enough to follow the recommendation."

*

Dr. Ju's Journal—14—Late Summer, 1970

The Doctor is under stress from all directions. It is not amusing. Sick people are very demanding. You must give them part of your life force to help them heal. They need it—some more, some less. But the doctor must learn to protect himself, or pretty soon nothing is left to cure new patients with. Worn out.

That is why I do many small exercises to make energy—exercises that I learned from the monks. Rub fingers through hair. Bathe face with dry hands. Rub Shen Men points together on the wrists. All the time, I do. And I speak to the students about; but do they appreciate the need for protection? Partly. But as students, they cannot really understand the sucking of sick people—or how terrible it feels when a patient will not get well. That takes a lot out of a doctor, even if he protects himself.

To do the doctor is only one side of the Five Excellences, of course. We who have a propensity, a talent, for healing think medicine is elevated; but this is not really true. A cultivated person must study and practice the other four every week—or how could you remain cultivated? Poetry and painting for refinement, calligraphy for communicating with beauty, martial arts to build a healthy body so you can live long enough to understand the Tao, and medicine so you can heal your friends. Those are the Five. A cultivated human contemplates the beauty of all nature. He is not a barbarian, burning and destroying.

Five Elements	HUMAN BODY					NATURE					
	Zang	Fu	Five Sense Organs	Five Tissues	Emotions	Seasons	Environmental factors	Growth & Development	Colours	Tastes	Orientations
Wood	Liver	Gall bladder	Eye	Tendon	Anger	Spring	Wind	Germination	Green	Sour	East
Fire	Heart	Small intestine	Tongue	Vessel	Joy	Summer	Heat	Growth	Red	Bitter	South
Earth	Spleen	Stomach	Mouth	Muscle	Meditation EXCESSIVE THOUGHT	Late summer	Dampness	Transformation	Yellow	Sweet	Middle
Metal	Lung	Large intestine	Nose	Skin & hair	Grief & melancholy	Autumn	Dryness	Reaping	White	Pungent	West
Water	Kidney	Urinary bladder	Ear	Bone	Fright & fear	Winter	Cold	Storing	Black	Salty	North

Chapter Five

Techniques in Gwa Sah & Moxa

1. Acupuncture points are transducers of energy.
2. A transducer changes one form of energy into another.

"There are many ways to stimulate an acupuncture point," Doctor Rosenblatt said. "Needles can be used. Burning Moxa which creates heat. Electricity. Massage. We even use lasers these days.

"The purpose of all these techniques is to start a spark. That spark actually changes the flow of the meridian, changes the nature of the energy by activating it.

"The acupuncture point is a group of pacinian corpuscles (or perhaps Krauss end bulb receptors, which look about the same). In any case, these bulbs contain liquid crystal structures that act as transducers, converting an incoming form of energy into another more healing form of energy. The Chinese call this changing biologic energy "chi."

"Is the energy already contained in the bulb?" I asked.

"I don't think so," the Doc answered. "The bulb is a transducer. One form of energy goes in and another comes out. As an example, when a crystal is squeezed, a measureable electrical charge is released. This is called the piezo electric effect. The needle squeezes the bulb, thereby creating a spark at the transducer that allows a more healing flow of energy."

"But let's talk for a minute about Gwa Sah and Moxa. Dr. Ju showed us these two techniques that stimulate superficial flow—energy flows that aren't connected to major meridians, but are the network of minor meridians on the surface of the skin where the *wei chi* flows. The wei chi is the defensive energy that initially

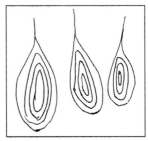

Kraus end-bulb

protects the body from invading influences. The first line of defense."

"In Chinese massage techniques, the wei chi is stimulated by rubbing the muscles and the connective tissue (fascia) between the muscle layers. Heat from the practitioner's hands loosen the tight muscles and promote the flow. At a deeper level, the healer sends healing energy into the patient's muscles. All these surface techniques are focused on undoing the knots in muscles that create a blockage in the energy flow.

"Massage is one technique, and Gwa Sah is another. Gwa Sah works more on the blood. It is said: "When the chi moves, the blood flows. When chi is blocked, the blood becomes stagnant."

Gwa Sah is based on pulling the trapped blood out of the muscles, raising it up to the surface dermal layer where it is washed away by the body's circulation. Traditionally, a small piece of jade, which had been lubricated with a medical oil such as calendula oil, was used to scrape lightly over a muscle spasm.

"A muscle that is in spasm traps blood in the capillaries by clenching up. Because the blood isn't flowing through the muscle in a normal manner, the muscle becomes locked and rigid, and therefore painful. The Gwa Sah technique pulls this locked blood out of the deeper capillaries, and brings it to the surface where it is reabsorbed. New blood can flow into the muscle and the block releases. Balance is restored."

Kathleen Rosenblatt had just come in from running an errand. Hearing that we were talking about Gwa Sah, she said, "Dr. So (that's James So, Tin Ya, head of the Hong Kong Acupuncture College) used Gwa Sah on me while we were studying in Hong Kong. I had developed a mild asthma, I think because of the dampness. Hong Kong, situated where it is around a large harbor on the South China Sea, gets a lot of rain and it's wet most of the time. He scraped the jade across the muscles between the ribs on my chest until I was striped with red welts like a red zebra. It hurt like crazy. I was screaming in pain, but he just kept on scraping, totally disregarding my pain. The Chinese are generally very stoic people. I guess they just decide to disregard pain. They burn Moxa sticks right on the skin down to the ash, something we never do.

"After Dr. So came to Los Angeles to work with us at the UCLA Clinic, he was living in our guest house. I noticed one day that he had moxa scars covering his back. You have to be very stoic to tolerate that."

"Martial artists train themselves to disregard pain," I said.

"Maybe," Kathleen said. "I wonder how they do it."

"Why would anyone want Gwa Sah treatment if it hurts that much?" I asked.

"It usually feels good on the back and neck, but the chest is much more tender. I'm way less harsh in my treatment that Dr. So is. I've treated you with Gwa Sah," she said. "You know."

In fact, I did know. My shoulders are generally semi-bound up from typing at my computer. I guess I must hunch over. On several occasions Kathy has treated me with Gwa Sah when my shoulders were killing me. The scraping technique feels good to start with, but as the number of scrapes increases exponentially it starts to hurt. The pain is this side of unbearable, or nobody would have it done to them. But Gwa Sah really does work. My shoulders felt better, and there is no pain at all once the scraping stops. Kathleen tells me that my experience is completely avoidable. "If a patient is more sensitive and the scraping is causing pain, they need to tell their practitioner who will ease up on the pressure or use a more gentle hand massage until the spasm improves. It's never supposed to be that painful. Men often don't speak up because they think it shows weakness," she added, with a knowing look,.

*

Dr. Ju's Journal—15—Late Summer, 1970

To be the doctor, you must feel like you are the one who can cure the ailment. You. Not your teacher, not the more famous doctor in the next town, not even your friend who is in practice with you. But you. And here is where the large ego comes in. Without the confident smile in your heart, you are lost.

We are not a doctor with high toxic pills, hoping and praying that poisons will cure this patient. We are not faith healers. No, we are more like master electricians, repairing the electric circuits.

And like a good electrician, people hear about you. Word of mouth is powerful for good work. An example: I got a letter yesterday from the Commissioner of Policemen on the island of Tahiti, inviting me to come visit his tropical paradise. While I am there, he would enjoy me to treat himself for an ailment that nobody can fix, and also treat all his policemen. He would be honored to pay for my ticket and hotel, and a nice roll of pocket lettuce. Well, well, electricians are *needed. I'm not totally sure that I am honored to treat policemen; but I guess I am. Policemen are people, too. And the Commissioner has the symptoms of jaw pain that responds very well to acupuncture.*

I will hopefully seem like a very smart electrician.

I wonder what they drink in Tahiti? Coconut wine? Ha, ha. Anyway, I think I will go to Tahiti. My students would probably take delight in a vacation from me.

*

"To show the contrast in the two techniques, acupuncture is point, point, point, opening successive gates in the deeper energetic sense—the other, Gwa Sah, is used to promote the flow in the outer defense energy. They are both very important in maintaining health.

"Another aspect of Gwa Sah is that it pulls heat out of the body. The patient needs to keep the area that has just been gwa sahed warm and covered, so that no draft invades the area, or the treated muscle may slip back into spasm. Because of this need to keep the freshly treated area free from drafts, Southern climates are favored. Dr. Ju came from Canton Province, which is quite southern and warm. Gwa Sah is not used so frequently in the cold northern climes, like Beijing."

*

Dr. Ju's Journal—16—Winter, 1970

It's strange, on Tahiti and the other nearby islands, the people are worried about their immune system. Really! Nowhere else that I have ever been are people worried about building immune. Other places worry about kidney chi, or keeping the monkey (male organ) strong, or a heart attack. It's because on Tahiti they know they were downwind from the nuclear bomb tests at Bikini Atoll and the Marshall Islands. They saw what happens to people who are downwind, and they are worried.

I worked all two weeks treating the police, who are nice guys. They like to drink Scotch, not fermented coconut. I treated their wives and children and grandparents. Everybody. But I'm not sure I did it right. Nobody knows how to do medicine for this. Not really.

We were really stupid to do those atom bomb tests.

And I did have one truly good success. The wife of the Chief of Police had a condition called uterine prolapse, where the ligaments get weak and allow the uterus to somewhat fall down onto the bladder and vagina. This is painful and more than a little frightening to the woman; but it is a condition that usually responds quite well to acupuncture treatment. Except in this woman's case, no improvement was noted as I treated.

Then I had a tweak of insight, like a blast from the past, as my students are fond of saying. I remembered a line from the healing chant that my masters made me memorize. It translates something like, "To tighten the falling: burn moxa cone middle of the chest." Middle means on the mid-line, halfway between the nipple line and the supra-sternal notch.

I had never understood this part of the chant. It had never made sense to me; but there it was, clear as a page from a textbook. And it worked like a charm. The wife of the Chief of Police responded just like the rhyme said she would. Her prolapse started to cure overnight—amazingly, it just sucked back to where it was supposed to be. She began urinating out much of the fluid that had built up in her body from this condition.

I treated her every day using this one point, and by the time I boarded the airplane to return to the USA, she was almost like a young girl again. It was like a miracle, even to me! How did I remember that jingle from so long ago?

*

MOXA

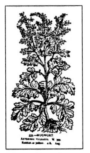

Artemisia Vulgaris plant (Mugwort)

"*Moxibustion* is a technique to provide concentrated, deep-acting heat at the exact spot where it is needed. Moxibustion gets its name from the herb, moxa (mugwort) which burns in a very consistent, controlled way so that the physician can apply heat to an area without burning the skin. Moxibustion actually brings energy (chi) into the system, because it burns at a particularly beneficial frequency of radiant energy, of which heat is only a part."

"How does it do that?" I asked. I'd been treated with moxa several times for muscle pulls and found it to be extremely pleasant. It operates on the borderline between pain and pleasure, much like certain Chinese cuisine, for example, Tang-Tang noodles which are so peppery hot that they numb your lips, but are so delicious that you can't stop eating.

"An acupuncture point acts as a transducer," the Doc said. "It transforms the heat energy of moxa into body energy. A transducer changes one form of energy into another. It is said that moxa brings new energy (in the form of radiant energy) into the system—needles don't. Needles open channels and rebalance. Moxa stimulates.

"Moxa is the dried fur-like underside of the leaf of the Artemisia plant, commonly known as Mugwort" Dr. Rosenblatt continued changing the subject from Gwa Sah. "The plant grows in China and widely in temperate climates. I've grown it here in Los Angeles. After harvest, it is hung upside down to dry. When dry, the leaf is crumbled in a strainer. The leaf part turns to dust, but the fur part balls up into a cottony clump. Then it is packed into a cloth bag so that air can circulate when it is hung up to age. Interestingly, Mugwort is often found in the wild growing next to poison oak. It acts to prevent poison oak skin rash if it is rubbed on the skin before contact. It's surprising that we often find plants growing near each other in the wild that have interactive properties.

"After harvesting it is still considered to be "green moxa" for the first two years, but as it ages the cottony substance becomes brownish in color. It takes three to five years for proper aging.

"We have a bag in the storage room that has been aging for twenty-five years. It was grown and harvested in 1974. The older it gets, according to Chinese medicine, the better the control of the burning ember is. If mature moxa is burned on the skin, the heat doesn't sear the surface. It penetrates.

"Moxa is considered by the Chinese to be non-poisonous, that is why they use it for heat, as opposed to other herbs that burn.

"In one medical formula, moxa is mixed with small amounts of several other herbs and is packed into a cloth or paper tube. This is called "pole moxa" or a moxa stick. The end of the pole is lighted and as the ash forms, the even heat is held near an inserted acupuncture needle. Warmth from the burning moxa is transmitted down the needle—into the body right at the acupuncture point. This technique is called "Indirect Moxa." It is warming, and promotes flow of blood and chi, thereby removing blockages.

"In "Direct Moxa" a ball of moxa cotton is rolled into a small cone and burned directly on the skin. The primary reason for using direct moxa is to alleviate intense pain and generalized cold conditions, like menstrual irregularities, which result from lack of energy (yang deficiency) which causes the yin to become excessive.

"Sometimes direct moxa is burned directly on the skin on a powerful point on the centerline of the abdomen, just below the navel called, the "tan tien" (CV 6) to increase yang energy—but most practitioners are currently wary of these direct techniques because of the ever present threat of law suits if scarring should occur.

*

"A few years ago we had three cats" Dr. Rosenblatt said, relaxing into story mode. "Two calicos and a black, all from the same litter. One night, when they were still little kittens, somebody stepped on the black cat. It was an accident. The black kitten was impossible to see in the dark.

"We nursed it back to health by feeding it with a bottle. But when it started to eat solid food, it would choke. One night, after the cats were a little more grown, I found this cat out in the front yard, choking to death. Literally. Choking on canned cat food. I turned him upside down, massaged his belly and the food popped out.

"I took him inside and Kathleen held the cat down while I burned moxa on a slice of ginger on his throat, and another cone of moxa on a fresh ginger slice on top of his head. One treatment and he never choked again. We had that cat for many years"

"Most people don't have fresh ginger in the refrigerator just waiting for an emergency," I suggested.

"True, but most people aren't acupuncturists. Ginger is a well-known medicinal plant. As a platform for burning moxa, it's soothing. It makes the treatment much more yin. Moxa by itself is very yang. The cat needed yin energy, not yang."

"Another time, Kathleen and I were vacationing in Mexico, when I got an attack of Montezuma's Revenge. I was really sick, vomiting and diarrhea, even thought my time was up. Then I remembered a moxa technique for food poisoning. Fill the navel with salt, and burn a cone of moxa on the salt."

"Just regular salt?" I asked.

"Yes. Salt from a saltshaker. I had Kathleen help me since I was really weak. I rarely get sick, but I was that time. We always travel with needles and moxa, of course. She broke off a piece of moxa stick and lit it on the bed of salt. As my navel warmed up, I started feeling better. The protocol is to keep burning moxa cones until you hear the stomach rumble—then burn one more. We did the treatment three times that day, and the next day I was totally well. We went to visit some Aztec ruins that we had wanted to see. I feel totally lucky to have learned all these techniques and tricks from Dr. Ju and Dr. So. I can't even imagine what my life would have been without their teachings."

And I can't imagine what my life would have been like if I hadn't met Dr. Rosenblatt. Round and round it goes, from teacher to pupil. Direct transmission of knowledge. How many years has Chinese medicine been around? Several thousand years, at least. Long enough to get a few things right.

***

Chapter Six

Five Aspects of Energy

We were seated one evening at the sushi bar at the stage of dining called "filling in the corners" when I asked the Doc if there were any serious, solid, laws of energetics.

"Acupuncture is the study of the laws of the movement of energy in the body," he replied. "As energy moves through the body, it obeys certain principles, just as electricity has its laws in a wire. For instance, Ohms Law is E=IR (voltage equals current times resistance). The Power Law is P=IE (power equals current times voltage). So too in acupuncture we have laws.

"To begin with, there are five aspects (or functions) that energy must support in a living system. These five aspects relate to the movement of energy."

Assimilation
Transformation
Transportation
Accumulation
Elimination

When you know about these five aspects, you know about energy. At least, how it is in humans."

"How about the first one, then," I asked. "Assimilation."

Assimilation

"Our body is not a self-contained organic system. It needs to absorb at least four kinds of food from the environment.

Solid Food
Liquids
Air
Impressions, the input to our senses.

"Solid food. To maintain and repair itself, the body needs a ready supply of amino acids, which form the complex molecules for tissue building. Therefore, the brain control center tricks the mouth into thinking that food tastes good. After we fall for the trick and eat a bite, the internal organs (mainly the digestive track) refine and adjust this raw material to feed replacement cells. If the food we gobble down lacks a mineral that is necessary for a building block, we suffer for it later with improperly maintained cells.

"Water. The body is 93% water. We're kind of like an inland sea, awash in the fluids we drink. These fluids, primarily water, provide the medium to dissolve salts and crystals, as well as acting as a lubricant and coolant for the body.

"Water itself has several unusual properties that have to do with magnetism and energy. The water molecule (H_2O) is an atom of negatively charged oxygen with two atoms of positively charged hydrogen hooked on.

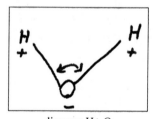

diagram H+ O

"In a healthy state the angle between the two hydrogen bonds fluctuates (since it is an unstable bond) in such a way that it becomes a resonance circuit, like a tuning fork, responding to certain beneficial frequencies in the environment. For instance, every high school chemistry student knows that surface tension of water swells after exposure to a magnetic field. I've also seen surface tension alter dramatically after exposure to the hands of a healer. This shows that water is responsive to electrical/magnetic stimulus. Water stores information imparted to it as frequencies in the angle between the hydrogen bonds.

"In illness, however these hydrogen bonds become almost horizontal, making no angle to resonate with incoming frequencies.

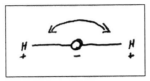

Diagram flat water

"Like any energy source (magnetic in this case) water gets used up in our system. Therefore, of course, it is necessary to replace the old demagnetized water with new water on a daily basis."

"My grandmother thought that drinking gallons of water during illness helped elimate the bad germs."

"Flushing is important," the Doc said. "But it's probably just as important to absorb really fresh magnetized water. Migratory birds use fluctuations in the magnetic field to orient themselves on their journeys, why shouldn't we?"

"How about the air we breathe?"

"Air. Along with oxygen, our lungs breathe in any and all substances in the air. For instance, energy fields might be in the air."

"Oh," I said. "Like the atmospheric orgone that Dr. Reich was researching?

"Wilhelm Reich was one of the giants," he said, letting more emotion show than usually. "It's a real shame that he wasn't better understood."

I knew that Reich had been hounded pretty hard during his life, but innovators often have that honor. People miss what they're aiming at.

"One of the absolute giants," the Doc restated. "Reich's discovery of the orgone accumulator was a brilliant advancement. It was a layered box of alternating organic and inorganic (metal) layers. He found it would build up a charge of what he called orgone energy, which is atmospheric energy that surrounds us all the time. In much the same way that a battery composed of two dissimilar metals accumulates electrical charges, the orgone box gathers and accumulates the energy that surrounds us. This is a basic principle of energy assimilation.

"The red blood cell with its inorganic iron core and protein coating is actually an energy (orgone) accumulator. Not only is oxygen transported to every cell, but this is the exact mechanism which assimilates atmospheric energy into the body, carrying it to each individual cell. The red blood cell

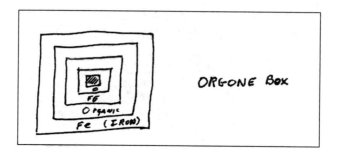

is astonishing, really.

"The oxygen and energy fields in the lungs become a type of food to feed the red blood cells, which in turn recharge the other tissues. And, of course, all the great teachings agree that proper assimilation of air is critical for the transmutation of course food into the finer food for the higher centers."

Transformation

Once the body takes energy in, it transmutes it into a usable form. This phase is called Transformation of Energy. Food is broken down into component nutrients—sugar (glucose) is transformed in a tiny part of each cell (mitochondria) to produce precursor ATP—the energy currency of the cellular level. Vitamins in food act to promote chemical actions in the body. Many chemical transformations can't take place without these essential vitamin catalysts. Water that we drink lubricates the joints and linings of organs and vitalizes all the cells, which are seventy percent water.

A molecule of air contains not only oxygen, carbon dioxide and nitrogen, but also a tiny, measurable charge of pure energy. Then we breathe air, this energy charge is attracted to the hemoglobin in the red blood cells in the lungs, where it attaches to the mitochondria mentioned above, thus charging the red blood cell with bio-electricity.

Oxygen and these energy motes act on the glucose to produce ATP (adenosine tri phosphate), which we spend to fuel the cells. Cells perform at maximum levels when they get enough ATP.

The sense organs take in impressions such as the light of the sun, or rock music. These are transformed into simple electrical signals, which pulse in an energy wave heading from the sense organ (eyes, ears, tongue, skin) to the central nervous system (brain and spinal chord). When an impression comes in, it doesn't stay pure. For instance, I see and hear and taste at the same time, and these incoming impressions wash into each other creating layers of increasing complexity.

A simple sense impression would be the knee jerk reflex that happens when your doctor bongs your knee with a rubber mallet. The sensation travels along one input nerve, affects one level of the spinal chord and sends a message along an output nerve causing the knee to jerk without the participation of the rest of the spine or brain.

This is simple, but other impressions and sensations can integrate to vastly higher levels of complexity as they rise up to the brain. Imagine the taste of licorice or the narcotic effect of coffee. Layer upon layer of experiencing.

To make this even more complex, imagine the impressions that are already in the brain from previous stimulation. These older impressions flit back down the nerves to mix with and influence the newly arriving impressions.

One of the higher aspects of transformation is the creation of eggs in females and sperm in males. This is the highest level of ordinary human transformation of energy. The sexual dance is about bringing these finest sex energies together for procreation.

It is said that monks and holy hermits use this sex energy for self-development.

Transportation

In order to make sense of these incoming waves of energy, the body is arranged so that these energetic waves can be pumped to receptor sites in every organ and cell of the body. This pumping is how we transport the incoming energy (made of food, air and impressions) to make it available to use for our daily activities.

There are three highways for transporting energy and nutrients. The largest and most commonly thought of road is the *blood vessel system,* which moves oxygen, food nutrients and atmospheric energy that has attached itself to the hemoglobin.

The second highway is the *nervous system,* which transports sensations from the sense organs to the central nervous system (brain & spinal chord) where they are analyzed and categorized so that we can make sense of these impressions. This is a high order of magic, if you think about it. How really do you know your fingers are drumming on the table? It could easily be your toes instead. Only the amazing computer of the brain and spine makes sense of it.

The nervous system is a two directional highway, like any real highway. Moving one way (incoming) are sensory (afferent) nerves bringing their message to the brain. Motor nerves (efferent) carry the return message back to the muscles, which contract as a result of this stimulation causing the body to move. On this highway, bio-energy moves strongly through the neurons and slows at the synapses.

Some movement is automatic. You don't think about the movements of your intestines or the dilation of your blood vessels when a blast of alcohol hits them, but these are also controlled by the efferent (motor) nervous system.

Other movements are voluntary. You can decide to lift your arm in the air, and simply do it. This is also possible because of the nervous systems.

The third highway involves the most refined energy—this is the *meridian system*, which is so fine that many people don't believe that it exists. This system is the fastest of the three highways because it is made of pure energy, and in a way it directs the other two energy systems with its overriding blueprint matrix function. And it is interactively responsive. This is all very remarkable—almost inconceivable—because these three highways work together to balance the system. Perfect health, perfect balance is the goal that every living system strives for.

Basically, when raw material moves from one energy level to another, this is transformation. For instance, when a bank robber becomes a priest, this is a kind of transformation—although sometimes the boundary is blurred between saint and sinner. Our cells, however, have no trouble telling when there is enough glucose and oxygen in the mitochondria to form ATP. When there is enough ATP, the cells are happy and energetic, and so are we.

Accumulation or Storage

Since we are not reptiles, we need to maintain a temperature that is usually higher than our surroundings. Maintaining this temperature takes a lot of energy. And movement takes even more energy; therefore we need to store energy to draw on when we need it. To accomplish this there are *accumulation sites* in the body—such as the liver which stores glycogen (used when sugar levels drop—sugar is burned to fuel movement). One problem of modern

Western life is that we store too much.

Fat is a classic storage mechanism for storing fuel to use in lean times. Due to the abundance of most Western diets (at least for the affluent) storing fat around the belly is a fact. Native societies (where we all came from) experienced feast or famine. Making it through a hard winter was a life threatening experience century after century. Storing fat became a survival strategy. The people who survived and therefore passed on their genes were genetically predisposed to quickly put on fat for later use. Humans are kind of like bears in that way. Storing fat is good, if you have to live off it until spring.

The spleen is another organ that stores bio material to use later. The spleen stores red blood cells for times of stress when the tissues need more oxygen. Like fat cells, the spleen can over-store. In extreme cases this can cause disease, and the little organ must be removed. Fortunately, spleen energy is still there, so balance can be achieved.

Each meridian has a storage point, called a *xi point*. These points are like a reserve in your checking account that can be tapped when you are otherwise depleted. These points are used by an acupuncturists when the system is low in general energy and there is no strong meridian that can transfer the energy. Like if your kayak tips over in chilly water and you can't get it righted. If you stay in the cold water for long, the system uses up all of its reserves of heat (energy) and a possible treatment at the time of rescue would be to stimulate these points.

The storage area for incoming impressions is the brain. We call it memory. We can relive experiences by recalling an event. For example, recalling an emotional experience stimulates your heart rate—sometimes even more than the original event. Embarrassing moments can be relived practically forever.

Elimination

With transformation completed, all the energetic juice is squeezed out of the nutritional raw material. The residual is eliminated as feces and urine. This is waste for us, but it makes food for plants, which then make food for us in a circular system we call life on Earth.

In the same way, O_2 is transformed by breathing and then expelled as CO_2, which is breathed in turn by plants as a primary food source for photosynthesis. Plants use the carbon element (C) as a food source, and expel O_2 as a waste product. The simplicity and staggering complexity of this dance between plants and animals gets more amazing the deeper one looks.

Elimination of the vibrational impressions from the senses takes the form of day-dreaming and normal dreaming during sleep. So many of these impressions enter the human system in the dullest of times, that they either must be used up by super awareness, or they must be eliminated like other food, so that there is room for fresh influx of new impressions.

Dr. Ju's Journal—17—Spring, 1971

They wake up from their nodding off to sleep when I talk about the monkey (male organ) and the monkey terminal (female organ). So I talk about it often, maybe too often. The boys like it better than the girls. They try to receive it studiously and take notes.

But it's important. Besides being interesting, proper sexual knowledge does not grow on trees. You have to find somebody who knows. If I, their adopted father (ha, ha) who has studied these matters exhaustively—purely from the medical and longevity point of view, of course—if I don't tell them about the monkey to keep them from falling asleep, who is going to?

"You have to be careful with the monkey," I tell them. "When monkey gets together with monkey terminal, it weakens kidney."

Which, of course, is true. They maybe don't believe me, but at least they wake up.

"Now, you are young and strong. Can put monkey to work with monkey terminal two, three times for one week. But later, you be old. Only can do one time. Kidney get too exhausted."

They smile sheepishly and do not want to believe. But later, when they do get old, then they will believe.

Must have strong kidney, or live life always fearfully. Kidney strengthen from doing T'ai Chi. This I also tell.

Chapter Six

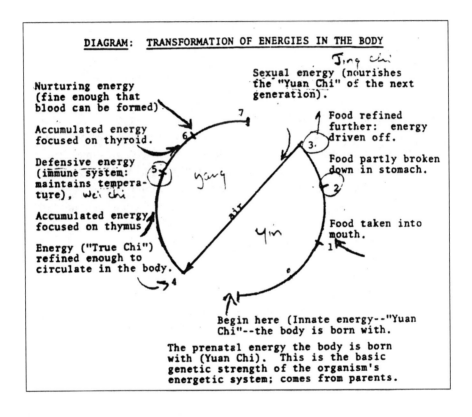

DIAGRAM: TRANSFORMATION OF ENERGIES IN THE BODY

Nurturing energy (fine enough that blood can be formed).

Accumulated energy focused on thyroid.

Defensive energy (immune system: maintains temperature), Wei chi

Accumulated energy focused on thymus

Energy ("True Chi") refined enough to circulate in the body.

Sexual energy (nourishes the "Yuan Chi" of the next generation). Jing chi

Food refined further: energy driven off.

Food partly broken down in stomach.

Food taken into mouth.

Begin here (Innate energy--"Yuan Chi"--the body is born with.

The prenatal energy the body is born with (Yuan Chi). This is the basic genetic strength of the organism's energetic system; comes from parents.

Chapter Seven

The Yellow Emperor, and More

The origins of acupuncture are shrouded in the mists of time. One might say that this art was an accidental discovery—trial and error in a warrior society looking for ways to heal fighters. Most discoveries in every field happen in the context of a researcher at least looking in a specific direction. So posit a group of very intelligent Taoist monks living in the high mountains of China, whose purpose in life was to discover what is actually true about humans and Mother Nature. Suppose this group of fellows and girls asked the question, "How does this astounding phenomenon of the body curing itself actually happen?"

Legend has it that these monks had time to look at things as they are because many of the old Taoists lived to be 150 years old, so they really did have time to investigate items of interest. As these inquiries became more talked about inside the Chinese monastery system, eventually an adept acquired the ability to see auras, or see deeply into the body, and with that ability "saw" the meridians and the spinning vortexes of energy at the junctures of the points. Then began the task of explaining it to his friends, and making sense of it all.

With that as a backstory, the long history of Chinese medicine has had many illustrious practitioners, and virtually all of them were Taoist monks. The entire field grew directly out of the Taoist monastery system, where this specialized knowledge was passed on from master to disciple for three thousand years. This is long enough to develop a few healing modalities, if you're trying.

Chapter Seven

Dr. Ju's Journal—18—Late Spring, 1971

I like to feel the energy. Most people walk with their palms sideways, beside their legs, but I walk with my palms downwards, bent at the wrist so I can catch the energy of the Earth as it presents itself to me on the small wind of my walking. The exact middle of the palm is very receptive to this free energy gift. And of course, receiving this energy into the body, especially for a doctor, is very rejuvenating. I say rejuvenating because to do the doctor means to give your life energy, a little or a lot depending on the patient's need. Healing, of course, is about energy exchange. A doctor weak in energy might send the patient to buy herbs from the herbalist, letting the energy from the little herbs do the healing. That is okay. The patient is healed. But the strong doctor—strong in his life energy—can cast the needle to the exact energy vortex that is deficient in energy. His energy animates the little surge that the needle makes at the acupuncture point to turn the patient's stale energy into healthy, flowing energy. That is why I walk with my palms down to gather the energy that I am going to need later in the day.

I think Howard understands this. Some martial artists are quite aware of energy in their hands. He is one. My UCLA Lo-fan students think that walking this way is peculiar. I see them making a bit of fun at their teacher's expense. Louie does. I see him from the corner of my eye. He is sensitive and could feel the energy, but he prefers to make fun. Ah, yes, not everything about the life of a teacher is flower petals along the path. One needs the patience of a stone Buddha statue, waiting for them to catch on. For the light of understanding to start to glimmer.

*

Sometimes the Taoists were in favor with the Chinese rulers and sometimes they weren't, but always they were regarded as the physicians of the country. Consequently, until the 20th Century revolution, they were left mostly unmolested to develop their medicine because it was needed. Also, having the luxury of an uninterrupted culture and uninterrupted language for all of those centuries was quite helpful to the long transmission that has become the Chinese system of medical knowledge, which includes acupuncture, massage, herbalism and energetic exercises. All of these techniques involve the use of bio-energy as a principle part of helping the body to heal itself—which was undoubtedly the original question perceived high on a wind swept crag in Hunan Province.

Their orientation centered on the concept that the energy flowing from Heaven and Earth influences the body in a harmonious way, and that the physician could assist in this harmonization by pushing the energy flow a little bit today, and a little more tomorrow. The main thesis was that both disease and death are related to a disharmonious flow of energy, but that health followed from harmonious energy.

That orientation still holds true today. We acupuncturists seek to establish a balanced, harmonious, flow of energy in the body—that is the end point. That is the goal. From the perspective of forty years of American Acupuncture it seems evident that Dr. Ju arrived in the new world of America with the specific task of transplanting a growing stem from a tree that was endangered. It may be that the West becoming so interested in the old Taoist's ways reflected them back like a mirror to the Chinese, so that they then began to reinvestigate their disregarded medicine after Mao's revolution.

*

Dr. Ju's Journal—19—Summer, 1971

I like the weather in Las Vegas. The dry heat is good for me. Makes me feel strong, cocky almost—and a doctor who is strong can cure people just by looking at them. Well, not really—I still have to place the needles.

Las Vegas people invite me to visit, twice a year like clock work. They like to be healthy. Free nice room—lots of wine and dine. Many patients. They almost form a line to see me. That's the way it should be.

I took a few of the students with me this time. It was amusing to see them starting to understand that a living can be made with these little needles—making people feel almost like new. And of course, at dinner time there was lots of opportunity for gum-boi toasts. Bottoms up with every course. This is good.

So suddenly we were all talking about why not get a legal license for Chinese medicine around this country, the USA—and start here in Nevada, where they love us. Some of the wealthy patients here in Las Vegas were even offering to help. Well, well.

I have to appear enthusiastic; but I'm not sure, at all. It's too soon, isn't it? The hospital doctors will eat us up, if we jump too soon. And these boys don't know enough yet. They don't know anything! How could they? I better take some of them to Hong Kong, so they can at least have a piece of paper degree. And that will take a year or two.

Chapter Seven

These new Lo-fan sons of mine are so darned eager—they're like a pack of hunting greyhounds. But they don't even bother to consult Stems and Branches to see when the appropriate timing is to be Earth shakers.

*

The truth is that nothing similar to the long uninterrupted stream of Chinese culture has ever happened in the West. It's not easy to explain why not. All original native cultures are very old, but let's just say that the Chinese have maintained their civilization for perhaps five thousand years, without being knocked off course by war, flood or calamity. They have been lucky in that they happened to control a very large area, so that volcanoes did not decimate their entire culture as happened to the Minoan civilization. Neither did tsunamis, earthquakes and glaciers ever destroy everything so that they had to start over from scratch. Instead, Chinese people have continued from generation to generation in a literate, if sometimes harsh culture, and the Taoist monastery tradition survived, the so-called heart of China. And the Taoists developed medicine.

Different doctors had to treat different diseases, so those cures were added to the aggregate. Someone would have a vision while in a meditative trance, and because Taoism believes in inclusion, the vision wasn't thrown away as crack-pot thinking, but was kept as a part of the mix. There was time and inclination to investigate almost everything that could be conceived of. The strong and the subtle were both regarded as equal parts of the practical energy question, because yin without yang is simply an unclear way of looking at reality.

But if Taoism was so dominant over the centuries, why has China developed with such difficulties—overpopulation, tyrannical rulers, political upheaval? The truth is that Taoism hasn't been overwhelmingly popular, ever, even though every Chinese person admits that Taoism is China. But it has been left alone—to evolve as one main ingredient in the stew that is China. And because Taoism was left alone, acupuncture and Chinese medicine could grow naturally—which isn't a straight line, but is a *spiral*—waxing and waning.

Over the long years, many different schools have been dominant inside the monasteries. Sometimes the Five Element people held sway, sometimes the Eight Conditions, some centuries it would swing over to Confucianism with his concept of right living. In the 20th Century the traditional medicine was largely eclipsed after the Sun Yat Sen epoch attempted to Westernize medicine. The Communist regime attempted to push traditional ways back to the forefront with the Barefoot Doctor movement, which admittedly was a pale echo of what medicine had been when the monasteries were fully flourishing. This movement sent many rather rudimentarily trained practitioners into the Chinese villages. They were somewhat equivalent to public health nurses here. Anyway, because medicine had broken down, these Barefoot Doctors were sent with a few herbs and one needle to areas where no other doctors would go. This was before the Cultural Revolution came to China, and its excesses nearly broke the system.

"Tradition asserts that the ancients were wonderful practitioners. Imagine that there are two spirals—one degenerating and the other accelerating. We in the West, caught the last gasp, the last few practitioners, and then we grabbed onto it and threw lots of money and new energy at it just before it blazed out of existence. The people of the world were very lucky, because modern Chinese doctors and politicians really cared nothing for the old ways, and would have let them pass from human knowledge. We were very, very lucky.

"That's what Dr. Ju was doing here. He was the White Crane! He was *the guy*! Dr. Ju's mentors and master teachers recognized that the West with its vitality was the hope for this type of medicine. For better or worse, we are the yeast of the *new* medicine. The hope is that this tradition can be slipped inside of Western medicine, really like yeast, and then a very nutritious loaf of medical bread can be baked. Healthful to all. Beneficial to all."

Dr. Ju's Journal—20—Summer, 1971

After a month of frantic activity of teaching and packing and making sure that my family was provided for in my absence, we finally got on the airplane for Hong Kong. Myself and two students: Steve, the Chairman, and Kathy. I had hoped for more students to take to Professor So; but these special two will suffice. The two are still not married, which makes an awkward situation; but if every situation didn't turn out to be awkward, it wouldn't be my life. Oh well. Many of the other students drove to the airport to wave goodbye, which was good. It is good to be a revered teacher.

Hong Kong is spectacular, as always. It is a city where a person can breathe freely. The rules are very clear. Nearly everything is for sale, therefore money rules—but not like in the US. Different. A million degrees of sub-

tlety. The money of a doctor is different than the money of a gambler. Not really, but yes really. It is quite remarkable as I pay attention to it through the eyes of my students. They are fitting in quite well. Quite bright Lo-fan. And after a slight disagreement over money with Professor So, they are enrolled and doing well. Near the head of the class. That Professor So is a pistol. I almost had to give him chicken feet, when he changed the fee we had agreed on. I am well aware that only two students came, but two is better than none, isn't it? It is teaching doctors, for Pete's sake, not belly dancing.

Professor So has quite a good college to get a piece of paper degree; but he is a Christian, raised by missionaries. He is very Chinese with good ancestors, but sometimes he appears to be a Lo-fan. Really, I came within a quarter inch of giving him chicken feet. I think Steve and Kathy noticed that I was blazing mad. He was dragging my face in the mud before my students. This anger I have to watch at my age. Weakens kidney chi much worse than monkey joining monkey terminal. Anyway, now is harmony, and we are visiting places, and eating real *Chinese food.*

I think I should move back here fairly soon. USA Chinatown is a very pale second place to this. But of course, my vision, my mission isn't finished yet. It is difficult to understand why the spirit world wants real Chinese medicine among the barbarians, but it evidently does—so I am here to serve.

*

"The secret goal that we were all involved in together, Dr. Ju and later, Dr. So, and all of the American students, was somehow to train enough acupuncturists and put them out into America like yeast. To make three dimensional bread, not flatbread. Really, there shouldn't be Eastern and Western medicine—there should only be *good medicine.*

The Yellow Emperor is a mythical character, who reputedly brought acupuncture to China, and as a side issue also invented political organization, writing and agriculture. THE YELLOW EMPEROR'S BOOK OF INTERNAL MEDICINE (NEI CHING SU WEN) is the classic in the field. The book first appeared in print about 240 BC. In those days, a person would write a book and say, "The Yellow Emperor wrote it in 1000 BC. By luck, I discovered it stashed in this honorable old trunk." The authenticity of age was probably good for sales.

Anyway, the Nei Ching was written as a dialogue between the Yellow

Emperor and his Prime Minister, Chi Po. It's a very philosophical treatise, filled with information about which acupuncture points to use at particular seasons of the year. "Were people healthier at one time?" asks the Yellow Emperor, in the opening paragraph of the book. "Have we lost a knowledge, or system of health care? Or is it that mankind is becoming negligent of the laws of nature?"

This was, of course, in 240 BC. Chi Po knew the answer to all the Emperor's questions. "In ancient times," he answered, "mankind understood and harmonized with the laws of nature and thus cultivated a healthy body. The people lived to ancient age without becoming dim of sight or weak of body." The book goes on to roll out the laws of nature and medicine which lead to a healthy body. But it proceeds from an important premise—how to maintain health.

The Yellow Emperor would probably be surprised at the surge of interest that the West is now showing in his three thousand year old tradition. Here in America, the ball started rolling in 1971 when James Reston, the Editor-in-Chief of the New York Times, burst his appendix in Beijing while doing the media background for President Nixon's trip to China. Acute appendicitis, of course, must be treated immediately, so there was no time for Reston to jump on a plane back to the States. He had to trust the Chinese. Naturally, they sent in their best physicians. And as a matter of normal Chinese procedure, an acupuncturist was employed to relieve his post-operative pain by using needles. Mr. Reston was quite impressed by this maneuver as well as with the Chinese surgeons who saved his life. Returning to the States, he devoted many New York Times columns to acquainting his readership with Chinese medicine.

At about the same time two prominent American physicians—Dr. Paul Dudley White, who was President Eisenhower's physician and Dr. E. Grey Dimond, the grand old man of cardiology, visited China. They observed acupuncture anesthesia being administered by needles in a complicated brain operation. On their return, they made no secret of being very impressed by this rustic practice—of 3000 years duration.

Whether the Chinese were as impressed with our tourists is a matter of speculation, but a small surge of public interest began in the United States, chiefly in the newspapers since Reston was very well respected by reporters, and also the medical establishment took notice.

In any case, Eastern medicine came out of the monasteries, and took a long-term approach. Prolonging life, rebalancing, treating chronic illness—because this medicine came out of the Taoist philosophy of life and how to live correctly. Life unfolds and develops in stages.

Western medicine basically developed in the Napoleonic Wars. It is based on European battlefield medicine, which is where surgery developed. As a result of the advent of cannon wounds which splintered bones, many amputation techniques were developed during this war. As a result, Western medicine focuses on emergency techniques—the quick fix, then getting the soldier back to the battle. Stopping bleeding, treating infection, keeping the patient breathing when breathing has stopped. This is the one area where the West really excels—emergency medicine. The Chinese talked about the circulation of blood and chi, in written texts from the 1st Century BC. They had very little surgery.

Even though Western medicine is fantastic in emergencies, Chinese medicine did discover ways of dealing with emergencies. In the next chapter, we will delve into a few of these Chinese First Aid techniques

* * *

Chapter Eight

First-Aid with Acupuncture

Here are a few unusual tips for things that go wrong with you're out camping or at the theater—or even at home.

1. When the Baby Doesn't Eat Well—there's a point inside the tiny middle finger's second crease. The second crease down, or up. It's the same either way. One prick of a needle at this point to draw a single drop of blood. Or take baby into the acupuncturist if you don't want to do the needling.

2. A sudden nose bleed—heat with a burning moxa cigar, or a tobacco cigarette at the point in the middle of the thumb joint, right above the thumb nail.

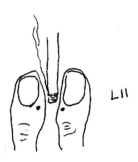

Heat the opposite thumb from the nostril that is bleeding. Careful! Don't put the burning coal close enough to burn the flesh.

3. Sudden episode of fainting—finger needle (fingernail). Use your finger as a finger needle on the point right in the middle of the cleft (philtrim)

in the upper lip. Direct pressure until you can feel the horizontal cleft in the underlying bone.

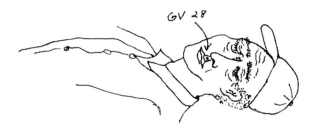

"We were never sure if Dr. Ju meant finger needle or if he didn't know the word for fingernail, or if he was using both concepts at the same time." Dr. Rosenblatt mused. "But actually that is exactly the kind of thing he would do, making a play on words like finger needle.

4. Headache (frontal)—Finger needle on the Hoku point (LI 4) midway at the juncture of the thumb and forefinger. Firm pressure on this point. If you have a headache, this point will be findable by its soreness.

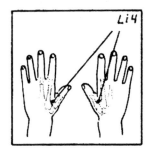

Most of the major acupuncture points are a little bit sore all the time. That's one way you can find them. A vortex of energy is going to have a certain sensation when it's pressed.

5. "How do you know if you're having a stroke?" I asked

"Strokes are caused by either a blockage in the blood flow in a vessel in the brain (ischemic stroke) or breakage in a blood vessel in the brain (hemorrhagic stroke)—but before that there was a blockage in the energy. "Where the energy flows, the blood goes," is the Chinese saying.

"The first step toward a stroke is an energy imbalance. Possible symptoms are paralysis on one side of the body. Difficulty in speaking or slurring words because one side of the mouth doesn't move is a frequent symptom of a stroke.

"Of the two kinds of stroke, it is said that the ones that happen in the morning when you get up is usually "blockage" type. Whereas stokes that occur during the day when you're exercising are more likely to be "hemorrhagic", because there is more blood flow and a blood vessel breaks in the brain.

"First-aid for both kinds of stroke is the same. Finger needle in the bau wei point (GV20), which is almost directly up from the high point of each ear at the center of the skull. At this point is a tiny indentation, smaller than your finger tip. Direct finger needle pressure downward at this point, hard. If an acupuncturist is present he will know where to use the real needle, otherwise do this finger needle technique until the patient comes around. Immediately get the person to the hospital. Many techniques have evolved recently for dissolving clots and stabilizing the blood pressure.

"Western medicine is terrific at stabilizing a stroke victim in ways that Chinese medicine is not so skilled. For instance, usually the blood pressure goes way down after a stroke. This needs to be stabilized by boosting the pressure. Tightening the blood vessels down is a very good way to increase the pressure in the vessel. Using a class of medication called pressors to increase blood pressure is used very successfully. Sometimes medication can be used to dissolve the blocking clot in the brain.

"Then in a day of two, the bruising that has resulted from blood in the brain or the oxygen starvation in the area downstream from the clot must be repaired or the quality of life will suffer greatly. In both of these cases hyperbaric oxygen chamber treatment infuses blood in the damaged area with pure oxygen, greatly speeding healing and the use of damaged limbs and speech ability.

"Acupuncture is a great help in stimulating the flow of energy which should promote collateral blood flow around the blocked and damaged areas, and in the case of hemorrhagic stoke, acupuncture promotes coagulation

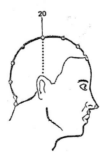

and healing of the wound. By and large, the drugs that attempt to do the same coagulation in order to patch a hole that is bleeding have many unwanted and undesirable side effects. Acupuncture becomes then, the treatment of choice for repairing stroke damage. This is a classic example of Western medicine being excellent at emergency stabilization, whereas acupuncture is the ultimate treatment for reorganizing health after a stroke. The best of both worlds.

6. Hiccups—can be cured with a finger needle right in the cleft of the big knuckle of the middle finger. Try it the next time you have hiccups and become a believer.

7. Nausea and Vomiting—feeling sickly, use finger needle at Pericardium 6. (Noi guam.)
"Strangely enough every point on every person is slightly different. Odd, but true. This point is two inches up from the inner wrist crease in both wrists, and it lies beside the tendon where it falls into a somewhat deep pocket. The point is *not* covered with muscular tendons, but is to the side and deeper. Once you find it, push with the finger needle (nail).

"Once I was visiting Mexico City to give a series of lectures, and I got the *tourista* due to something I ate. But I had to lecture anyway because all the doctors were waiting. All through the lecture I was finger needling this point like crazy because I was about to toss my cookies all over the podium. Surreptitiously, I was really leaning on this point, because I was seriously sick, no kidding. But this technique somehow got me through the lecture.

"Right afterwards, a doctor from the audience came up on the stage and asked if I knew any acupuncture point that could stop vomiting. Small world. So I suggested that he could rub and press on P6 right there in his wrist, as it had just saved my lecture from becoming a sideshow."

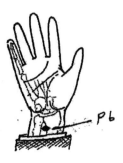

8. Testicle Pain (from trauma) A grounder bounces up wrong and chimes you. You're playing touch football and you're wife's heel happens to kick you right in the family jewels by mistake. You're rolling on the ground unable to breathe. The pain is astounding. What to do?

Here's the point to use. On your foot is a point called Kidney 2. Located halfway down the inside of the foot, right under the bone and tendon. Use your knuckle to deeply press on this point. Press in and rotate the knuckle around. The point is under the head of the first metacarpal.

Do it yourself? No way! You can't even breathe. But after you can breathe and when the stars and blackness start to clear away, stick your knuckle in this point. Or if a team-mate gets chimed, you could even help him out.

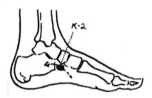

9. Imminent death (from shock, blood loss, heart failure). With some kind of needle-like instrument or sewing needle break the skin at the Ting points, which are the ending or beginning points on all five fingers of each hand, and all ten toes.

Break the skin of all six points on each hand and each foot. If you're out camping and can't call 911, what else are you going to do?

10. Drowning? While we're on the topic of serious maladies, how about drowning?

"These are real emergency points. Someone is about to die! These are last chance points. Midway between the scrotum and anus on a man, or between the lower end of the labia and the anus on a woman, is a sensitive little stretch of skin, called the perineum, where the starting point of the Conception Vessel (CV1) is located. In Taoist mediation this point is called the bottom of the sea. Stick a needle up to an inch deep for an adult, 1/4 to 1/2 an inch for a child.

It is said that if the drowning person defecates, he will live.

At the same time someone should do artificial respiration. If you're treating alone, try artificial respiration first. If it works, fine and dandy—if not, try needling CV1.

Having read this chapter, you will, of course, want to take an acupuncture needle with you on all future vacations, fishing trips, walks and even excursions like washing the dishes.

11. An attack of sneezing? You can't stop. Something got in your nose and won't go away. Finger needle the same point that is used for fainting, GV24. Also use LI20, which is on a line with the bottom of the nostril, out to the side in the fold of the lips. That line. The nasal labia fold, also called the Smile Line. Finger needle those points. Relief is in sight.

12. Diarrhea Out in the Mexican wilderness you get an attack of the runs. I told you not to eat the chili relleno from that pushcart. Wow! What to do?
Well, lie down. Take a thimbleful of table salt and fill up you navel. Slice a quarter thick slice of fresh ginger root. Poke ten holes in the ginger slice with a toothpick. Put the slice on top of the salt in your navel.
Make a little cone of raw moxa about a three/quarters of an inch tall. Set it on the ginger slice, then light the moxa cone on fire. It smolders without a flame, but you will see it burning. Let it burn down. If it gets too hot, take it off for a minute, then put it back. After the first cone burns down, blow off the ash from the ginger, light another cone and burn it down also. Burn three to five cones. When the treatment has been successful, you hear a rumbling in the stomach. Light one more cone after the rumbling sound in the stomach, burn it down, then the treatment is over. Most people experience one final fling of diarrhea, then the discomfort normalizes. Yes, we talked about this treatment earlier in the book, but it's worth repeating.

13. Vaginal bleeding (non-menstrual or very heavy menstrual)—A point on both big toes, dai-dun, Liv 1, above the toe nail, midway to the first toe knuckle. Make a cone of moxa and burn it right on that point. Take it off when it's too hot. Use 3 or 4 cones. The bleeding will slow down and stop.

* * *

Chapter Nine

Layers of Disease

"The first stage in a disease process," Doctor Rosenblatt said, "is a change in the body's specific frequency."

"How can you tell when you get a change in frequency?" I asked.

"You can tell," he assured me. "We have hundreds of words to describe it. I feel out of sorts. I feel unbalanced. I feel like I'm coming down with something. Something has changed in me. I feel weak. We're not exactly feeling the frequency change, but we're getting sensory input that the frequency *has* changed. The result of this change is that we get a sour taste in the mouth, or excessive fatigue or something like that.

"This is the stage of self-help. Nobody runs to the doctor at this stage. What they do is eat some Vitamin C or chicken soup or go to bed, something to make themselves feel better. A good thing to do is a Tai Chi exercise called A Prayer Wheel which actually brings fresh energy into the body."

"What's that?" I asked.

"I'll show you one of these days," he promised. "Anyway, if the self-help fails, the disease enters the *Latency Period*. This phase is when people should see a practitioner/doctor/healer. They need help from the outside.

"An old Chinese saying applies to the latency period, "The superior physician treats a disease before it actually manifests." Almost every day I treat a patient for a disease he doesn't actually have yet. "Watch your large intestine," I tell him. If he watches what he eats, he won't get sick. Another example is the patient who comes to see me after he has been to his family doctor. "He ran me through a battery of tests; upper GI, lower GI, and he couldn't find anything wrong," he says. "My doctor said it must be psychosomatic; but I don't feel crazy. Something's wrong!"

"You do have a little deterioration in your liver," I tell him after checking the pulse. "Actually, it's in the energy that supplies and animates the liver. Let's see if we can fix you up." It's astounding, but the *"superior physician"* really does need to recognize disease in the two early phases, before it gets inside the fort.

"When the body is able to fight off the disease process, or is aided by the proper therapy, the disease will not progress to a deeper level. Then the *healing process* begins and the disease moves out of the body in the reverse direction that it moved in. The rule is: Healing moves from the inner layers toward the outer. A diagram would look something like an onion."

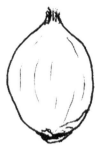

"No, not like that. Like the layers of an onion."

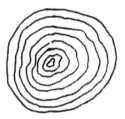

An onion - cross section

"A disease moves in through the layers and moves back out again to full health."

"Hey," I said. "That's really true! A cold moves just like that. You get a chill, then your nose starts running, and then you get a cough. When you start feeling better, the cough goes away, then you finally stop blowing your nose, and you feel great again."

"Just what I've been talking about," the Doc said. "There's nothing mysterious about it. If you get proper treatment when the disease is on the outer layers, it goes away a lot sooner—without leaving scars.

"It's the same in chronic disease which has worked its way inside due to no treatment, or poor treatment. A patient comes in with chronic shoulder bursitis, for instance. He's had it for many years and it moved inside and damaged his large intestine. Why…? The large intestine meridian runs down the shoulder and arm. Or perhaps the large intestine, itself, has caused the bursitis. Who knows which came first, the chicken or the chicken salad? As I treat the large intestine organ, the patient will almost always experience pain in the shoulder. He experiences the symptoms in reverse order from deeper to the surface.

"There's even a six point Law of Cure that illustrates the disease process exactly. I gleaned parts of it from an 18th Century homeopathic text by Samuel Hahnemann. A cure follows these six points:

Law of Cure

1. The system responds to disease by making the best possible response it is capable of at that moment.
2. Disease progresses from more external to more internal.
3. Disease generally progresses from upper body downwards.
4. As the body acts to cure itself, the disease progress will move from inside toward the outside. (note: Thus skin disease should seldom be suppressed for it is often internal disease moving outwards.)
5. As the body moves toward a cure, it will experience the same sequence of symptoms in reverse order.
6. The progress of cure will generally move from lower parts of the body upwards.

*

Dr. Ju's Journal—21—Winter, 1971

Sightseeing is fun and rewarding in Hong Kong. Opportunities for trade and business are always appearing. The Tan-Ka boat people living in the harbor are an example. Many families will spend their entire lives living on a boat. American people find it so interesting to live on a sampan boat in a crowded harbor. Quaint. But to us it is natural. It's like having a big truck for hauling freight in Los Angeles. Here the sampan hauls freight across the harbor, and maybe up the coast, and the family who is the crew lives on it. Normal and simple.

There are many fewer layers of law on the harbor water. Trade in all manner of items flourishes. Like a fish. How could officials make a law for a fish? He would swim away. Besides, I always really love Tan-Ka food. And occasionally drinking tax-free Johnny Walker is also enjoyable.

* * *

Chapter Ten

Causes of Disease

"So if the body desires to be healthy, why do we get sick so often...?" I asked the Doc.

"There are four major causes. Let's refer to them as the *primary causes* of disease. The first reason that we get sick is *inborn weakness*, which of course is a genetic weakness, possibly passed on generation to generation due to a defect in the Jing Chi (sex energy). This results in a lowered body defense at the specific area where the weakness is. Also, toxins present in the parents may cause inborn weakness in the child. Mothers who stop drinking and smoking, and try to eat correctly during pregnancy are, naturally, attempting to give their child a healthy body, but the toxin levels at the moment of conception would logically have to be factored into the whole picture, somewhere.

"*External factors* also cause disease. They're the *second* primary cause. Climatic conditions such as heat, cold wind, dryness and wetness seek out a weak point and enter the body. Then we also have to contend with radioactivity and noxious vibratory rates such as micro-wave radiation and fluorescent lighting. And people still fall off bicycles and smash up their cars."

"And some people catch a fish hook in their ear," I added.

"Right. You'd be surprised how many ear infections are caused every year from fish hooks." This was high sarcasm. There aren't that many fish hook injuries.

"The *third* primary cause of disease is *Emotion*," the Doc continued. "Our strong negative emotional reactions throughout life cause imbalance and blockage of energy at physical locations. These recurring emotions lock up the positive energy and won't allow it to flow. When you get angry, for instance, you can feel it affecting you, can't you…?"

"If I ever got angry, I suppose I'd feel it," I lied. "Luckily, I don't."

"Some people do get angry, though, and they stay angry. Or they find themselves in stressful situations, or they get sad or dejected. A lot of diseases are actually caused by emotional distress. I think most ulcers are. And probably most colitis. A large part of cancer seems to be emotional blockage, and maybe all of asthma is emotional.

"The *fourth* primary cause of disease is something simple, *diet*. We eat tons of crap in America and the West. Some places in the world, of course, people don't have the luxury of stuffing themselves with mountains of sugar and white flour and red meat. But in these countries, too, improper diet causes sickness. Lack of food, not enough calories, or mineral and vitamin deficit, can make you as sick as too much food, maybe even sicker.

"In addition to excessive salting of the good food we do eat, we now allow the food industry to add all kinds of chemicals to prolong the shelf life of their products. These additives are kind enough to pickle our innards when we eat them.

"Of course, most of our meat is fed toxic antibiotics and growth hormones. And our grain and fruit is sprayed with poison pesticides. Even the fish are poisoned by waste dumping.

"And if that isn't bad enough, we also ingest toxic substances from the environment—chemically polluted air, crap in the drinking water. Actually, we're subject to all kinds of hazards. And you even used to smoke!" He said to me.

I hung my head in shame.

*

Dr. Ju's Journal—22—Winter, 1971

Well, I am back to my home in the USA. It is good to be back, which makes me surprised. My second home, I guess. I am comfortable here, after all.

A China man can be invisible in the US. Amazing really. Even a doctor. Bill has driving me around to different parts of LA, and to UCLA. I can take a walk around and nobody notices. Nobody sees me. I am like the gardener, even if I always wear a white shirt and tie. I could probably rob a bank in most parts of LA and nobody would even realize I was there.

I got a letter today from Dr. So, thanking me for bringing my students. The Chairman and Kathy both were a credit to me and the US. Well, well. He wanted me to send him some more students. Perhaps. We'll see.

And I am teaching the students somewhat deeply about herbs. They have a flair for it, and they can categorize thousands of items. It is perfect for an herbalist. We walk in the hills around Los Angeles and gather plants. Quite fun and refreshing to be out in nature. It is so easy to get wrapped in city things and forget about trees and little plants. Very foolish to forget nature. Everything comes from nature.

The Chairman and Kathy got back two weeks before I did—complete with their Doctorate of Oriental Medicine from Hong Kong. Already they are planning to open an acupuncture clinic at their UCLA. They, the Chairman, Bill, and David, one of my Class Two students, have started a medical association, the National Acupuncture Association, it is called. Very important sounding and national. Why not international, I kid them. It is very dangerous, and also exciting to give young men a diploma. They often take advantage of the situation to push their new credentials around. And naturally, they wish me to be on the treating staff at their UCLA clinic—although I have no paper credential. This Clinic actually might happen. Many talkings and dealings.

But it is nice to be back in the USA. It is a different kind of excitement here.

The other day, I showed them the herb for amoebic dysentery that my masters taught me about. It was growing in a yard down the street from my apartment. I think it was accidentally just growing there, but perhaps somebody planted it. I got kind of excited and loud talking, which is out of character for me.

There has been many times in China that the amoebas get into the water supply. Perhaps they are always there. I believe that is why we drink the tea, because it is boiling the water. But sometimes the amoebas win. They get in the mouth, they get into the stomach. They do their very bad work. And nothing normal will put them to rest. But this little herb, this little plant with silky leaves and such a thin little stalk that you think to yourself that it will never survive until the next time we need it—this little plant gift from the spirit of the planet can make the amoeba flow right through and not stop to set up housekeeping. Amazingly wonderful. This plant has perhaps saved China people from being extinct. And there is was, growing right down the street on the way to the dim sum restaurant. Chinatown is such a remarkable place. I am surprised very often. And to most US people Chinatown is simply invisible, like an empty spot on the city map. Or at least, I think so.

Chapter Ten

*

"There are a couple of *secondary causes* of disease," Dr. Rosenblatt continued. "*Germs* and *microbes* or what I call bugs, are around us all the time; but they only march in when we're in a weakened state from one of the *primary disease causes*. It's really somewhat improper to consider bacteria and viruses (bugs) as the cause of disease in the strictest sense, because that view ignores the underlying energy imbalance.

"The *second* secondary cause of illness is *improper medical treatment*. One major form of improper treatment is the *suppression* of a previous illness through indiscriminately prescribed antibiotics. As I've mentioned, antibiotics have a strong tendency to drive a disease deeper into the body, where it lies dormant to spring up at a later time. Antibiotics can be used to successfully treat the acute manifestation of a disease and are often life-saving but one must remember to also treat the underlying cause. And replenish the good bacteria in the gut by giving probiotics after the course of antibiotics.

"An even greater improper treatment is called *iatrogenic disease* (drug or doctor caused illness.) This can be the side effects of any drug. Terrible cases of this kind of thing are being reported all the time. Everyone knows about it, but they keep swallowing pills. A couple of simple examples are bleeding ulcers caused by taking too much aspirin. Or puffiness and tissue breakdown caused by improper use of oral cortisone medication. I'll tell you a story about cortisone," the Doc said, wincing.

"I'm all ears," I replied.

"Many people who get iatrogenic diseases are wealthy, because wealthy people can afford to be over-treated. This woman was no exception, a very wealthy lady who had arthritis and back problems. She'd been given cortisone shots and prednisone for many years. Finally, she noticed a tremendous weakness overtaking her body. Her eyes started to protrude slightly. This went on for a year or so, at which point her doctors diagnosed hyper-activity of the adrenal glands.

"Cortisone, of course, is an enzyme from the adrenals (adrenal cortical steroid.) She'd been filled up with this chemical for many years and it caused an over stimulation of the adrenal glands, which is called Cushing's Disease. Her doctor's remedy for the Cushing's Disease was to wheel her into the operating room and lop out her adrenal glands. It's not funny, it's sad! Now she has to stay on cortisone for the rest of her life, because her body doesn't have the capability to produce natural cortisone. This was a medical blunder. If they pump in too much cortisone, she gets puffy. If they don't pump in enough, she gets tremendous pain all over."

"And you can't help her..?"

"Somewhat. I'm trying to limit the breakdown of her other systems. Some of these so-called medical treatments are unbelievably difficult to undo."

"That one was," I agreed.

*

Dr. Ju's Journal—23—Spring, 1972

The doctor is a professional, but he also has a calling. Is it a business? Well, that is a question, isn't it?

The Taoist monk is required by tradition to take care of himself, not to live by begging alms. And so it was decided that for a certain period of each year, the monk would go out from the monastery to practice healing, which he was allowed (and encouraged) to charge money for, to support himself and the monastery.

Healing is not a religious activity exactly, unless you might want to consider healing as a good deed that can add to the three thousand good deeds that are required. But not being primarily spiritual, medicine can be charged for.

But this Western tradition of making vast sums of money for being the doctor, even I find that disconcerting—and I am not a monk. Far from it. True, I had the great good fortune to find myself in a position to study the Five Excellences before the ancient ways of teaching were severely damaged by the hoards of young boys. But I do not despise money. Trading goods and services for goods and services is an honored tradition, am I wrong? But still. If you take the money, you're supposed to work hard to cure the patient. That is what the calling is about.

* * * * *

SECTION 2

THE PRACTICE

Chapter Eleven

Techniques for Diagnosis

I wanted to get the Doc's views on his diagnostic procedures. I've been visiting his office for years, so I'll first give a patient's observation of an office visit.

When you walk in, you get to see the receptionist right away. She's inside a big half-round window with no sliding frosted glass. She's right there. On the first visit she gives you a medical history form to fill out.

The form has several pages full of mysterious questions like has your handwriting changed recently. When I filled in the form, I thought it was smart to joke around with the more amusing questions. For sex I wrote yes. After I got to know the Doc, I found it didn't much matter what I answered. He's looking for different clues than a normal physician. The answers, coupled with your posture as you limp into his interview room gives him a general picture of your health. If you skip in, or do cartwheels, he kind of relaxes.

The Doc wears a white coat and a tie because most patients want a medical man to look medical. "If I was an African witch doctor," the Doc says, "I'd wear the correct feathers and colored paint. One has to look the part for the society one is treating."

He told me a cute story about a woman who came in and sat primly in the interview chair. He looked at her medical history form and saw her name was Mary Smith. "Hello, Mary," he said.

"You may call me Mrs. Smith," she replied, formally.

Somewhat surprised, he said, "Fine. You may call me Doctor Rosenblatt." This is an example of nimble medical repartee.

After looking at the form, he asks a non-directional question such as,

"What seems to be the problem? How can I help you?" Besides listening to what the patient says, he also listens to the *tone* of voice, which holds many clues to relative health. Harsh or weak, tense or relaxed voice tones signal underlying patterns of health in the body. For instance, anger shows as an imbalance in the liver. Excessive joyfulness may be an imbalance in the heart. Then with all this input, he works out an *energetic pattern* as quickly as possible.

"What is it about the energetic pattern that helps you diagnose?" I asked.

"Pretty simple, really," he replied. "I had a patient in yesterday with a chronic bladder infection. She first got the infection in 1990, so for fifteen years she's had to urinate day and night. It was also complicated by chronic yeast and trichimona. And she was also constipated. I started seeing a problem of sluggish movement of energy along the Large Intestine. Metal (lungs, large intestine) was not feeding Water (bladder, kidney). That's a rather normal blockage.

"I put together a hypothesis of her energetic pattern. As she told me more facts, I added them to an imaginary matrix (pattern) along which I assemble data. I form a graphic picture of what's out of balance, since the whole body is interrelated. Starting with a trial hypothesis, I lay down the facts to see if they fit a rational treatment. By putting the symptoms into a pattern, I arrive at a diagnosis.

"There are four basics basic techniquest for diagnosis in Oriental medicine:

LOOKING—seeing which leg is dangling.
LISTENING—to the voice (and maybe the odor)
ASKING—getting the history.
PULSES—in the wrist.

"For myself, I add a fifth set of diagnostic techniques if needed, electronic diagnosis: Kirlian photography, the Acuscope and radionics.

"After I form a mental picture of the ailment, I have the patient go into a treatment room and put on a gown. Then I take the pulses. Placing my finger tips on his wrist, I move over the twelve pulses until I complete my picture of the relative strength of the pulse from each organ."

"My thought about the pulses is that they're a way of getting me into sync with the patient almost psychically, so that I'm picking up on each specific organ at its specific pulse point." The Doc placed his finger tips on my right wrist as he'd done many times at the office. "At this point," he said, pressing with the index finger, "I'm looking for Metal. At this position is the Tri-heater. It's almost like dowsing for information."

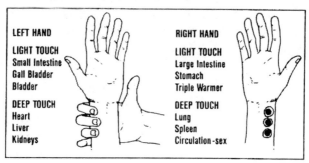

Old Chinese wrist pulse chart

"The Chinese describe the pulses as sensations at specific points on the wrist being transmitted to the physician's fingers like the tension on a bowstring. Diagnosing is a very subtle art. Pulses are extremely subtle sometimes, and sometimes not."

"Tell me what actually happens when you stick an acupuncture needle in somebody?" I asked.

"Well," the Doc said. "I start with a general treatment the first few visits, trying to move energy through the circuits. Many people are so affected by just a general flow of energy that their problem is alleviated. On the other hand, some patients are so identified with their ailment that even when their system is virtually healed, they still have arm pain, for instance.

"'Hey, I feel much better, Doctor,' they tell me. 'My constipation is pretty normal now and I'm able to make love to my wife for the first time in years, but my shoulder still hurts. I'm not sure you're doing any good.'"

I smiled, knowing I'd said much the same thing.

"A person can be going to his regular doctor for ten years and isn't being helped, but that same person expects miracles from acupuncture. If I don't completely cure his problem in two visits, he starts telling everyone that acupuncture doesn't work.

"Here's a Law: THE LAW OF ALTERNATIVE METHOD

Any alternative method must be much more effective than the generally accepted method to be considered of value.

"And since acupuncture *is* very effective, people keep coming for treatment," I said.

"Right. In the case of the lady with the fifteen year old bladder infection, she'd been treated with antibiotics for at least ten years. In fact, she'd just come off a course of strong antibiotics which proved ineffective, that's why she came to me. Two things had to be done. One: her body's resistance had to be built up so the bugs wouldn't keep invading. Two: the inflammation in the bladder and the urinary tract had to be reduced.

"I started with some general points along the Large Intestine and Bladder Lines. One needle beside the knee, one beside the ankle, one in the fork of the thumb, trying to smooth out the flow of energy between those points. Then I used two needles below the navel on the Centerline Vessel for general energy, because once I get the circuits open, I want to pick up the general energy level.

"That was it for her first treatment. I asked her to return in a week. Next time I'll work up a homeopathic remedy for her. But I want to see how her system is responding first. Maybe she'll need a stronger treatment, or electrical stimulation from an electrical device, or maybe heat from moxa, but I have to see how she is before I know. In a sense, acupuncture is like an art form because today's treatment depends on the effect that yesterday's treatment had on the system. It's interactive, just as all living things are interactive.

"In Western medicine we have a binary (yes and no) system. Did that remedy work? No. Try this one.

"Acupuncture, however, is interactive. How have the symptoms changed? If there's a change along one line, I want to push it toward balance. I'm constantly reassessing the treatment each time I see the patient."

House Calls

My first patient had trigeminal neuralgia, which is an inflamed nerve in the jaw. It's one of the most painful things that can go wrong. The constant sharp pain keeps the sufferer from eating, kissing their spouse or doing much of anything. They live in fear of another pain attack. And it responds poorly to Western Medicine pain control treatments.

This woman's husband called Dr. Ju on the phone pleading with him to please help his wife. Dr. Ju handed me the tray of needles and said, "Your patient." He told me the acupuncture points to use and worked up a treatment scenario.

I went over to the woman's house in a trailer park. She was in terrible pain. Her doctors had operated on her several times with no pain relief. They injected her nerve with alcohol in an attempt to kill it. Finally, they had taken out a part of her cheek bone. Nothing helped.

I put needles in the points that Dr. Ju had shown me, and within a few minutes the pain dissipated. I arranged to see her in a few days to check on her pain.

The next day I told Dr. Ju the whole story. He was very complimentary, which of course stroked my ego. It was wonderful to be "doing the doctor." This woman and her husband were life-long clients, coming to see me every few years.

*

A woman I just saw today is now ninety-four years old and a holocaust survivor. She was hidden in an Austrian convent, pretending to be Catholic, and never went to a camp. I have been treating her and her sister, who is now one hundred and two, for a number of years. Both are amazing, energetic, women with a real zest for life.

Ten years ago, I was called by a neighbor to make a house call to Trousdale Estates to treat this woman's older sister, who was 92 at the time. I didn't particularly want to go. I was busy and their large house was way up in the hills, but her neighbor's dad was a friend of mine, so I went.

I walked into the foyer. The woman met me sitting in a wheelchair. She was a very engaging woman, but told me she was paralyzed from the waist down. Her doctors at a major teaching hospital, not UCLA, said the paralysis was caused by a stroke in the spinal cord. The spine is a part of the central nervous system, which also includes the brain.

I did a series of acupuncture treatments with electrical stimulation on the needles. After the second treatment, she was able to stand. After a few more treatments, she was walking and even driving her car up until she was nearly a hundred.

Sadly, the elder sister passed away last week at age one hundred and two. She was bright and alert until the last few months. I treated her weekly for years. Even the last week of her life, she walked around her patio with her walker while I was there. Not bed-bound, but active until the last days. The younger sister is still bright and active, living on her own at age 94. Remarkable women.

Chapter Eleven

*

Dr. Ju's Journal—24—Summer, 1972

The calling of the doctor is from the heart to make another person feel better. To make the disease go back, and the health come forward. To bring the good energy in and push the bad energy out. To make the people of your little village glowing with healthy. This is the doctor.

The UCLA Lo-fan princes of medical administration have responded to my Lo-fan students and to the Chairman, who now has a OMD (Doctor of Oriental Medicine) degree. They all want a clinic; but the administrators want to control the rules. They want to pay me somewhat for my time and expertise; but they want to control the agenda, as they say. They, of course, know nothing about Oriental medicine. I and my students know acupuncture, but the administrators *must control the agenda.*

I worry that an extremely gigantic hospital and University like UCLA may not know about this thing called a "calling".

The monks that I learned from did not have an MD degree. They did not have a degree at all, but they came from a very serious lineage. The lineage kept people who did not have the calling out of medicine. Something to think about. For many centuries, the Taoists regulated medicine rather successfully, awakening the heart of the doctor.

Does UCLA, the very giant hospital do this method? I don't think so. But neither do the current Taoist monks—not after the hoards of sixteen year old boys swept through the temples all over China with their axes and butcher knives, chopping down the lineage and the sacred groves.

So now the lineage wants to grow at UCLA. Well, I know this is a good thing; but I worry about the calling.

* * *

Chapter Twelve

Homeopathy

The Doc asked in passing if I knew anything about homeopathy.

"A little," I said. "Those pills you gave me when I stepped on a dead bee at Venice Beach, and another time when I had hemorrhoids."

"It's absolutely vital stuff," he said, handing me a paperback book by George Vithoulkas. "This book is the most readable text imaginable. Without homeopathics I'd really be handicapped in treating."

I read the book by Dr. Vithoulkas called *The Science of Homeopathy*. It's a wonderful book based on exactly the same laws of energetic cure that the Doc talks about. Homeopathy was literally discovered in 1755 by Samuel Hahnemann in Germany while experimenting on himself using Peruvian bark (quinine). Although he didn't have malaria, the ingestion of Peruvian bark gave him all the symptoms of malaria. Quinine, of course, cures (or suppresses) malaria. Hahnemann developed the theory of homeopathy during these experiments (A hair of the dog drives out disease) and spent the rest of his life proving that his theory was a true healing premise.

THE LAW OF SIMILARS

"Any substance that can produce a totality of symptoms in a healthy human being can cure that totality of symptoms in a sick human being."

As opposed to allopathic medicine (Western) which works by encapsulating a disease with an antibiotic and driving it inward, homeopathy works by driving the symptom outward and expelling it from the body. The theory of exactly how this is possible is perfectly detailed in Dr. V's book. The Doc and I recommend the book.

*

Dr. Ju's Journal—25—Summer 1972

What do I mean when I tell my students not to write down notes? Yes, no note taking at my home and in the office. In the classroom, okay to take notes, because it is only theory. But in the medical office, you observe treatment, or you assist with treatment, so no note writing. This is practical, although the students want to rebel. Learning must go direct to the remembering place, that way nobody can take it away from you.

"I give you something that cannot be taken," I say, and sometimes I have to say it very firmly, because some of them are determined note takers.

Note taking is BS, as they say here in America. What if all your knowledge is scribbled down in a book, and what if somebody comes along and takes your precious book? I suggest this could happen, and they look at me like I am a crazy man. Who would want to steal a notebook with jottings about medicine in it?

If I had my knowledge of treatment written down in twenty notebooks and the thousands or millions of teen-age boys came running into town with the red book in one hand and a carving knife in the other like a swarm of bees, and no wisdom to temper the carving, what then? If that happened, you would run away, perhaps leaving your precious notebooks behind. And then you would not know how to be a doctor without your notebooks.

So yes, I say do not write down notes. Remember instead. In your heart and your mind, remember. I am not crazy. You are living in innocence of the deeds of your fellow humans. Or maybe your notebooks might burn up in a fire, while you are eating chicken feet at the dim sum restaurant. That is also something to think about.

*

"How do you arrive at a homeopathic cure?" I asked the Doc.

"There's one main method for diagnosing in traditional homeopathy," he said. "*Asking*. A traditional homeopath asks the patient pages of questions so he can isolate all the symptoms before he makes his first diagnosis. The more modern method is asking by kinesiology (muscle testing), the Voll machines, and radionics (electric feedback.) But homeopathy isn't the main thing I do. It's an adjunct for me. For better or worse, I'm an acupuncturist. I think in acupuncture terms. But sometimes I arrive at a supportive homeopathic remedy."

"Why...?"

"Because they really do work. I wouldn't mess around with them at all, except that they're energetic in nature. And they work."

"You can tell what's wrong with a patient by checking the pulses," I said. "You don't need to rely on asking for symptoms."

"Right. That's an advantage in diagnosing. It's not always easy to get the symptoms correctly identified just by asking about them. But neither in acupuncture nor in homeopathy is the actual symptom treated in the sense that it is in Western medicine. In Energetic medicine the symptoms are the key to the underlying energy imbalance."

"One thing that homeopathy pays a lot of attention to is *miasms*," the Doc reflected. "Dr. Hahnemann came up with that word to describe certain root illnesses that can be passed on through the generations. He was having problems in curing a variety of stubborn illnesses that seemed to respond, and then recurred. In depth research led him to these three root miasms:

ROOT MIASMS
Psoriasis
Gonorrhea
Syphilis

"These organisms, if not expelled from the system by the defense energy, can penetrate deeply into the body and result in total degeneration, ie, Cancer, Diabetes, Mental Problems, etc. And perhaps worse than the actual disease, a miasm can be passed on to unborn children in a form that may not give them the disease, but may weaken their defense system. Western medicine, in many cases, simply drives these organisms deeper into the body with suppressive therapies, exactly the opposite of correct treatment. Thus, the gene pool, which carries the hope for humanity, becomes successively weaker with each generation. A good homeopath is aware of the possibility of inherited problems and tries to expel the miasms before they become severe.

"So I use homeopathics or I don't depending on the patient," the Doc went on. "A woman came in the other week with a severe case of psoriasis. Her hands were encrusted with scabs and scales, and had been for years. She was recommended by a doctor friend of mine, who was at his wits end with her.

"Right away she started complaining about everything. She bitched so much that I came within a whisker of telling her I couldn't treat her; but she was my friend's referral, so I told her I was going to treat her with both acupuncture and homeopathics."

"What are homeopathics?" she demanded. "Are there side effects?"

"People are suspicious of doctors these days, but I told her, "No, it's not a drug." He laughed. "When I looked for the specific remedy I wanted to give her, I found we were out of it. I told her I'd order it, and she could have it on her next visit.

"She came back yesterday, and gave me another bad time. "Do you have to leave the needles in so long?" she cranked. But low and behold, her skin was the best it had been in twenty years. I decided not to give her the homeopathic after all. Acupuncture was working well on the level of the skin and deeper. Unfortunately, it hadn't improved her disposition.

"The truth is, it's not necessary to use all the different remedies at once. If I see that something is working, I continue with it.

"Homeopathy is relatively slow acting. A homeopath sees a patient every two weeks. It takes that long for the treatment to have its effect. In the acute stage of an illness, I see my patients every week, or twice a week or even three times if need be. But homeopathy is an important adjunct. Some people, of course, don't want to take pills of any sort, and with them I feel like I'm fighting their disease with one hand tied behind my back.

"A lady patient of mine suffering from sinusitis came in for a return visit. She handed the vial of homeopathic remedy I'd given her on her last visit back to me. "It's too sweet," she said, flatly. That was her final word on the subject.

"Okay," I said. I guess her sinus wasn't hurting badly, if she wouldn't do that much to help herself. "Come on," I kidded her. "Too sweet…? It's powdered milk. The lab has to use something to carry the drop of remedy on."

"I'm allergic to milk," she informed me.

"There's about three drops of milk in a whole vial of pills. But, hey, I can't hold somebody's nose and force the pills down their throat."

"I don't understand," I said to the Doc, "why the news media never mentions homeopathy when they're always talking about epidemics of herpes and AIDS. It can be such a breakthrough medicine that you'd think people would be flocking to it. I mean, it actually makes people well."

"There are very few licensed homeopaths in the USA," he said.

"What do you mean by that…?"

"There are only a few states that license homeopaths. If you have a license for some other medical specialty, you can practice homeopathy, otherwise you can't."

"That's absurd…!" I exploded. "It cures diseases…!"

"Maybe so," he said "But that's why you don't hear much about it. In Mexico and in Europe there are lots of homeopaths."

In spite of that, homeopathic remedies are now available in almost all health food stores, and in the medical section of most regular food markets. Most large cities have homeopathic stores with very large selections of remedies.

As we said in the last chapter, Dr. Rosenblatt occasionally makes house calls. I know it's unheard of in a big city like Los Angeles for a doctor to leave his office, but…. yes, Dr. Rosenblatt does sometimes. Maybe the fact that he grew up in Los Angeles, and rode his bike to baseball practice, makes him think that LA is his small hometown.

In any case, on a trip I made to Central California, I ate several restaurant meals and some fast food, and when I got home I was sick as a dog from food poisoning. Upchucking and the whole deal. In fact I was "flowing" from both ends. The next day it hadn't abated and I was really weak. I felt the end was in sight. I called the Doc and asked if he could come over because I was dying.

He dropped by before noon, put three homeopathic pills under my tongue and stuck a few needles in my knees and one or two near my navel.

"Ready for more pills?" he asked.

"Still have them," I said. The pills were undissolved under my tongue.

"Well, dissolve them," the Doc said. "How do you think they work…?"

I let some saliva dissolve the pills. He put three more in. I dissolved them, and pretty soon the daylight of healing let me know that I was on the way back to health. The Doc took his needles out and left me a vial of homeopathic pills called nux vomica. And there you have it, another successful house call.

*

Dr. Ju's Journal—26—Autumn, 1972

But no note taking has another deeper meaning, too, which is obvious if you think about it. Learning directly into the mind, the heart and the fingertips is

Chapter Twelve 119

essential, because these three must agree before healing can happen. Making a detour into note taking puts a Chinese screen between healing and the doctor.

Instead of note taking, the old time doctor monks decided to use mnemonic jingles like every school child uses to memorize the months. This is different than note taking, because it goes directly to the mind, where it can be instantly recalled—even if you're lost in the jungles of Borneo and need to perform a healing for dysentery with a few subtle points that you usually don't use. You forget the points, but a dim memory stirs that your teacher taught you these very points, years ago. So you go over the jingle—well, it's more than a jingle, it's more like a chant—and low and behold there is the cure for dysentery staring you in the face. It's in your mind, not in a note pad, which is lost in your office in Los Angeles, Chinatown.

But the very sad thing is that I know this chant, it is a part of my soul by now, but it is in Chinese, Canton dialect. I cannot translate it into American English. How could I possibly do that? The subtleties of this sing/song chant that comes down from antiquity are immense. I am no translator, I even hesitate to mention this chant to my students since I sadly cannot teach them. I think I must leave it in the hands of the Ancient Ones to send a translator if they want this chant to live on here in Hollywood.

*

"Disease exists in the body on several different levels. This is very important," the Doc said as we sat down at our favorite coffee shop reviewing our growing stack of notes. " The first indication of disease may be detected as a breakdown on the physical level, like the deterioration of an organ, bleeding, or infection. One must use the corresponding treatment methods to correct the problem *on that level*."

The Doc had raised his voice a bit to emphasize that this was important.

"That's why Western medicine is so effective at treating urgent and emergency conditions. Western medicine may utilize strong physical methods and what may seem to be harsh procedures in order to save a life. Deeper causal factors may have to be temporarily ignored in order to get the physical body back to a stable condition."

"But what about the deeper energetic factors," I asked. "How do they fit in?"

"The body is also composed of biochemical factors and, as you well know by now energetic factors," The Doc replied shifting into his professorial lecturing mode. "These three aspects of the living organism: (1) physical, dense, palpable tissue, (2) biochemical factors such as enzymes and hormones, and (3) energetic factors composed of flows of bioelectric chi. These three different densities, from the most dense to the finest, are all interpenetrated, one within the other. These three factors make up the living functioning organism."

Stopping for a moment to sip his coffee, the Doc continued. "You can see how each of these levels merge into the other. The dense, physical, structural matter is composed of biochemical factors, which are then composed of energetic (bioelectrical) factors in the form of charged particles. But each of these three levels are interpenetrated and interactively affecting each other. One cannot separate one density from the other without severely injuring or destroying the living organism."

"But the most important thing I want to emphasize at this point, is that when there is a disease state, illness or imbalance, the correct treatment for the correct level of illness *must* be used. If the focus of a problem is energetic then energetic methods must be used, such as acupuncture or homeopathy. If the disease is focused on the biochemical level then biochemical methods must be used, such as nutrients, supplements, or herbs. If the disease is focused on the physical tissue then more physical means must be used such as surgery or antibiotics."

Pausing for effect, the Doc continued, "Each level of disease must be treated with the treatment modality that is suitable for that level. This is the most difficult thing for new practitioners of any type of medicine to understand. They fail to realize that each treatment modality is a tool and each tool must be suited for its own job. My father would say, 'You cannot use a hammer to saw a piece of wood, or a saw to drive a nail'.

"And yet each practitioner thinks that their own form of medicine, which they specialize in, is the *only* modality to use on a patient. This is true not only of Western physicians, but also herbalists, acupuncturists, naturopaths, chiropractors and probably even Voodoo practitioners in Haiti."

"You know I think you're probably right about that," I murmured while trying to think of where I might find a local Voodoo man in West LA.

* * *

Chapter Thirteen

A Diet for 21st Century Foxes

I'd been listening to talk radio programs lately. Every host is compelled to have health experts on the program, because they always get a lot of call-in action from the audience. Audiences are very interested in their health. Every expert has a different theory that he's pushing. I find the conflict of opinion disturbing. "Do you know what's been bothering me?" I asked the Doc.

"What has?" he asked.

"Why does every theory about diet contradict every other theory? It makes me feel half crazy. I don't know what to eat, and what not to."

"It *is* pretty confusing," he said. "This fellow George Wilson did what I think is very interesting research on diet. It just happens to fit exactly into Oriental theory. Dr. Wilson analyzed the body to determine the acid-base (yin-yang) balance. He also tested the pH of urine after the intake of a wide range of food substances. He came up with his dietary principles through testing, and what he mainly found was that the food we eat seldom gets broken down properly due to the *combinations* we call a balanced meal. In my opinion, improperly broken down food is a real culprit. It makes sludge in the intestines and plaque in the arteries.

"It's important to remember that food is useful only if it produces and releases the energy necessary for the body to function on. Completely digested food releases all its energy. But partially digested food clogs up the system. Nutrient absorption is the job of tiny villi in the intestine. After years of bad eating habits, the intestines won't be able to absorb nutrients properly at all."

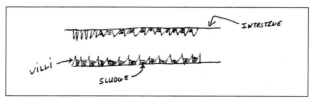
Villi in the intestine

"I'll get back to these villi in a minute, but first let's talk about the food groups and the enzymes which break down the food."

"There are five main food groups:

PROTEINS (meats, milk products, fish, nuts, etc.)
CARBOHYDRATES (grains, starches, beans, etc.)
NON-STARCHY
VEGETABLES (greens)
FATS (butter, oils, fat from meat)
FRUITS (apples, oranges, etc.)

"The problem in digestion is that each food group requires a different *enzyme* to break it down in the gastrointestinal system. Are you following this...?" the Doc asked.

"Fine so far," I said. "Where's the problem?"

"The problem is that each enzyme needs to be at *full strength* in the stomach and intestines to fully break down a food. When we ask the digestive system to produce more than one enzyme at a time, it doesn't have the ability to make these multiple enzymes at full strength. So the food passes through partially digested, if we eat more than one food group at a time."

"You must be kidding," I yelled, rather louder than I meant to. "Nobody eats only one food at a time, not even the Chinese and Japanese."

"You're missing the point," the Doc said. "I'm talking about the main focus of a meal. The Chinese eat mostly vegetables with a little meat. The Japanese eat mostly fish protein with a little rice, which is a simple carbohydrate easily digestible. Eskimos eat primarily pure protein, and stay young by rubbing noses. Here, take a look at this chart." He pulled a Xeroxed chart out of his briefcase.

"If I'm trying to cure a specific condition, or if a patient is seriously ill, I want the digestive system to work at its maximum. By eating food in the combinations suggested in this chart, you get the total energy from each food

Chapter Thirteen

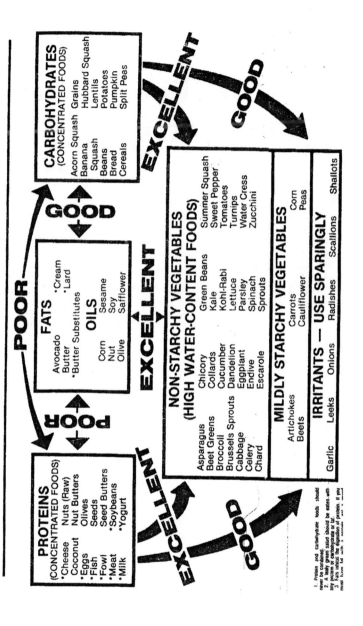

because the body fully digests it. Fully digested food is absorbed easily into the bloodstream and it doesn't sludge up the system."

"What about sugar...?" I asked the Doc. "Why isn't it listed on the chart?"

"I don't really consider sugar, natural or refined, to be a food. It's more like a poison. I didn't list any groups of poisons on the chart. There's no alcohol, no tobacco, no steel shavings."

"What does sugar actually do in the system that makes it so bad?"

"The worst thing it does is cause obesity. The high, empty caloric count is stored by the body as fat. Secondly, it interacts with bacteria in the mouth to form acid, which causes tooth decay. Thirdly, it over-stimulates the pancreas making it produce large amounts of insulin, which rapidly depletes the sugar causing the blood sugar level to drop dramatically (hypoglycemia). And if the pancreas is constantly stimulated, it eventually enlarges, which often leads to type 2 diabetes. This is a result of too much insulin in the system resulting in the body becoming insensitive to its own insulin. "

"I guess that answers my question," I said.

"As a rule of thumb," the Doc said, "*proteins* and *carbohydrates* should never be combined in the same meal, because they're complex foods and must be broken down in stages."

"I still think the American way of eating makes that almost impossible," I bitched. The thought of giving up meat and potatoes, chicken and rice, omelets and toast was suddenly very unappealing, even though I knew my digestive system wasn't really tip-top.

"I'm just laying out the ground rules for good health," the Doc said, mildly. "What anybody does with the information is up to them. To break down protein you need the enzyme *pepsin* at full strength. If the enzyme is diluted with liquid or other enzymes, the result in the stomach is a partially digested residue of protein called *proteinoid*. This proteinoid joins with fats to form cholesterol, which has gotten a lot of deservedly bad media exposure for blocking arteries.

"One of the initial enzymes responsible for carbohydrate digestion is *hydrochloric acid* (HCl). Diluted HCL results in *carbonoids*, which also join with excessive fats in our fat heavy diet, to make cholesterol.

"Fats, of course, are not evil in themselves, only when they combine wrongly, or break down partially themselves to form a harmful chain called a *tri-glyceride*. When the enzyme for fat digestion, *lipase*, is not potent enough due to competition with other enzymes, fat partially breaks down into *glyceride*. The glyceride molecules hook together in chemical bonds to form *tri-glycerides*, which make another type of sludge in the arteries. If there is plenty of lipase, then fats can be broken down into glucose (sugar)."

"Okay," I said, "Problems occur when we eat these several food groups at the same time. The stomach doesn't produce any one enzyme at full strength to totally digest any food. Instead of energy, we get sludge that mucks up the system. Everybody eats like that. That's why everybody is yucked up."

"That's part of it," the Doc replied. "Another poor habit is drinking vast quantities of liquid with meals. Everything from wine to beer to ice water, soft drinks, iced tea, coffee. Logically, all this liquid further dilutes the enzymes and makes digestion even worse. Liquids are good for people, but not too much at meal time."

"Makes sense," I said.

"Another thing is fruit. Fruit is terrific. It's high in liquid and roughage and, of course, fructose sugar, which of the sugars is the best. But when fruits are eaten with the complex food groups, it screws everything up. It adds one more enzyme, *fructase,* to the diluted enzyme stew. And the high water content in fruit further dilutes everything.

"Personally, I eat fruit no sooner than 30 minutes after a meal. You can tell when your stomach is ready to tackle a new food, if you pay attention."

"We skipped over salad stuff," I mentioned. "I guess you wanted to save it until last."

"Correct. Leafy green vegetables and all the non-starchy vegetables are the exception to the mixing rule. They can be eaten with any of the food groups, because they're *enzyme neutral*. In fact, they should be eaten in rather large portions because they provide roughage, and their chlorophyll-type water content lubricates the whole system. It forms a semi-soluble roughage"

"What exactly is this roughage that everybody keeps talking about..?"

"Roughage (from greens, whole grains) provides bulk in the intestines, which cleans the villi I was talking about earlier. Cleaning the villi is a very important function, because nutrients are absorbed into the bloodstream thru the villi."

"When we eat incorrectly, the sludge of proteinoids and carbonoids builds up around the hair-like villi and prevents them from absorbing nutrients. However, roughage rolls through the intestine and cleans the sludge off the villi."

"So eat lots of salad. A clean villi is a happy villi."

"If proteinoid builds up around the villi," I queried, "then proteinoid must get absorbed into the blood stream?"

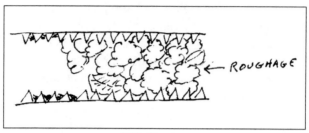
Villi Cleaning

"Exactly," the Doc said. "That's how plaque and cholesterol do get into the arteries. The liver, kidneys and the lymph system are responsible for cleaning this sludge out of the blood.

"The lymph system drains the garbage from the other systems. *Interstitial fluid* runs around between the cells sucking poisons out. The poison drains into various clumps of lymph cells, called lymph nodes, for cleaning. In the lymph node, infection is eaten by white blood cells. The lymph fluid drains to the kidneys, where toxins are filtered and expelled from the body.

But unlike other fluid systems, the lymph system has no pump. The heart is a muscle that pumps blood. The peristaltic system pumps the intestines. Spinal fluid is pumped by the movement of the spine. But the lymph system, which is crucial to the removal of toxins, is only pumped by *exercise*. That's one of the reasons why exercise is crucial to good health."

"I didn't know that about pumps," I said.

"You and millions of other people don't," the Doc replied. "But now you know. You're one up on the throng."

Dr. Ju's Journal—27—Autumn, 1972

I said to my students, "You come down to Chinatown this year and next year. See me. Watch me treat the patients. Learn to do the doctor. We will enjoy an important kind of fun together. I, the teacher—you, the eager student. This is the real fun that people can have with each other—learning, teaching about something important. This is the serious fun. We are having it together.

But after next year, you will do the doctor in your own office, with your own patients, with people you love who are sick. That is serious serious. Sick people need energy. You have to give it. And you can't get it back unless they get well. Money payment is okay, is necessary to live, but money can't really give back energy to you.

You give, you give, and soon you fall down deficient, not enough energy to cure, not enough even to make new energy. You are almost empty. Drained.

Ah, ha...! What you do now?

You think you can take some more lessons from me?

Well, maybe yes, maybe no. Maybe I will be gone someday. Move back to Hong Kong. Then what you do?

Well, you have to remember the secret inner parts of the Tao, and practice every day to cultivate your energy and awareness with Chi Gong and other measures. Then at some point, you will need a student of your own to teach, and the great serious fun can continue in an unbroken line.

* * *

Chapter Fourteen

Herbal First Aid and Dr. Ju's Arrest

Dr. Ju's Journal—28—Spring, 1973

My father likes it when I visit him. He lives in a cottage in the town of Fresno, California, which is a farming town. It's slow there, somewhat like village life in China. He moved to the USA when I was a boy because he could make money to send home, and the Great Land was not quite safe—and Taiwan was…an island. Fresno is somewhat like an island also, but we overlook that.

Before he left, he arranged for me to study as a day student at the monastery. My father was very prescient about my ability to do the doctor. He somehow arranged for the monks to test me for medical proclivity, and they agreed that I would make a good candidate. I slept at home, but had a work/study situation in the day, working in the kitchen, cleaning the main halls and courtyards in exchange for my lessons. And my father sent payments from Fresno. So I owe him for my beloved career as well as my life energy.

Now he is old and retired, but when he was in China, my father was a normal man, the manager of a small government office in Canton, who was caught in a revolution he certainly did not want. Anyway, he now lives in Fresno, and he likes me to visit.

He tells his friends that I am a doctor, the authentic kind, from home. So, of course, they have to stop over for a free treatment for their rheumatism when I visit his little town. I don't mind—my father had a difficult life. And I can help some of his friends to feel better, which is good.

Well, as it goes…the old people bragged of their healing to other people, and suddenly I am in demand in Fresno. I have to make once a month trips for treatments. Which is fine. I can use the money. It's gotten to be such big business that I have to rent a motel room to use as a treatment room.

And it's good practice for the students, too. Sometimes the Chairman drives me up north, sometimes Bill does. We have fun on those trips—I always try to tell them a few "whispered-in-the-ear secrets," to make them want to travel with me. It's very important for them to experience lots of different ailments—and there are some strange *cases out in those little towns.*

*

I stopped by the Doc's house one Sunday afternoon. He met me at the door with a large plastic fishing lure box. "Look at this," he said, excitedly. "This is probably the best idea I've had in a while."

"What is it...?" I asked.

He popped the lid open to reveal many one inch square compartments full of dried bracken.

"What is it...?" I asked again.

"Herbal first aid kit," he said, proudly.

"Really?"

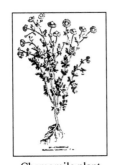
Chamomile plant

The Doc and I sat on the overstuffed couch in his living room. Placing the open box on a coffee table, he began explaining the merits of each herb.

"*Chamomile*" he said, pointing out some tiny yellow flowers. "Kathleen and I grow them in our home herb garden." I noticed that he had wrapped all the herbs carefully in cellophane to keep them from spilling over into adjoining compartments. "Chamomile is very good for stomach upset. Pour hot water over the blossoms to make a tea (or decoction). Drink it. Very settling for a queasy stomach."

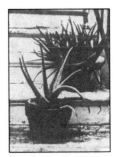
Aloe Vera plant

"*Aloe Vera*." He showed me two green spears of aloe vera, freshly cut and wrapped. "Especially good for cuts and burns. Smear the jelly on the skin surface. It promotes healing in an amazing way. Sometimes even a bad burn will heal with no scar, if you put this gel on.

"You can buy aloe vera liquid in a healthfood store, and keep a little vial of it in your kit, but I prefer the fresh leaf. We keep an aloe vera plant in the back yard. They grow quickly in the ground or in a pot, and

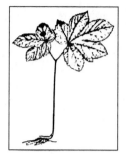

Goldenseal plant and cobwebs

provide handy first aid in the house. In colder climates, aloe vera can be grown indoors in a pot."

"*Goldenseal.*" He held up a packet of what looked like cobwebs, sort of. "Great for cuts and infections. It's a natural antibiotic, and the cobwebs make a scab that knits a cut together.

"Say you're out fishing on a half-day boat. The guy standing next to you makes a flailing back cast. His hook happens to snag your earlobe. After you finish cursing and seeing stars, you pull the hook out and wash the bleeding wound with fresh water, then you put a blob of aloe vera jelly on the cut and cover it over with a wad of goldenseal cobwebs. The goldenseal makes a very quick scab. Then if you haven't lost more than a gallon of blood, you can move away from the jerk at the rail and continue fishing."

"Do you grow goldenseal?" I asked.

"We could, but it's a pretty delicate plant. The easiest way is to buy it at a health food store or a Chinese herbalist."

"*Tobacco,*" he said. "Here's one advantage of smoking cigarettes." The Doc smoked when I first met him, but hasn't for a good 25 years, so I found the statement odd. But not for long.

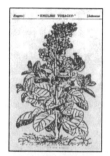

Tobacco poultice

He tore the filter off a cigarette that was in one of the compartments and squeezed the tobacco into the now empty compartment. "Tobacco is a good herb, as long as you don't smoke it," he commented.

"Imagine that our daughters are barefoot on the beach and one of them steps on a bee. Naturally, it hurts like crazy and she starts crying. You whip open the first aid box and make a poultice by wetting a wad of tobacco and taping it in place over the bee sting. The pain eases immediately and she stops crying, and you can breathe again. The main thing to remember about a bee sting is to get the stinger all out. When we get home, I'll give her a homeopathic called Apis Mel (Latin for honey bee), which is specifically for bee stings. What could have been a rotten day for everybody can be saved by herbal first aid.

"*Euphrasia* is another useful herb," he said pointing out some brown string-like twigs. "It's also called "Eye Bright" and is good for eye infections and things that get stuck in the eye. We make a tea out of it. The tea is good tasting and clears redness and minor eye infections. It can also be used as an eye wash.

TIME IS BRAIN

...a little story about euphrasia and other things.

The Doc was out of town for the week-end, and I was eating sushi for lunch with my family when, with no warning, a cloud appeared in the middle of my right eye. I attempted to wipe it away, assuming it was a tear, or something on my glasses, but the little cloud remained. It didn't seem life threatening, so I didn't mention it at lunch, although it certainly was off-putting.

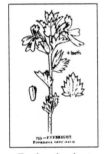

Euphrasia plant

I had very good medical insurance at the time, and an excellent eye doctor who I planned to call as soon as lunch was over. And my ace in the hole, Dr. R would be back Monday. I was a little worried, since a close friend was suffering a detached retina that didn't heal right, but I figured my medical team was tip-top.

The eye doctor looked into my eye with an ophthalmoscope (that instrument they use to look into the eye to see the retina) and told me that my retina wasn't detached. He sent me to an ultra-expert technician for further tests from an even bigger optic scope. They all confirmed that a tiny blood vessel had ruptured behind my retina. The cloud in my right eye would be a permanent feature of my vision. So I went to see Dr. R assuming he would fix it.

After the Doc had asked me all about the eye event, he had me lie on the treatment table and stuck a few needles in my knees and feet. Then he explained what had happened. The optic nerve forms a cup of retinal tissue behind the back of the eyeball. The retina is the end of the optic nerve, the only part of the brain that is visible with a scope that looks into the eye. I had had an infarction of the optic nerve behind the retina. An infarction is a blockage of the blood flow, usually caused by cholesterol. This blockage caused part of the nerve to die, hence the cloud, which was dead cells that blocked my vision, actually making a blind spot.

"Time is brain," is a catch phrase that every emergency room doctor knows, and few other people have ever heard about. "Time is brain" is specific to strokes and other maladies of brain tissue, like my eye. The quicker the doctor can restore the blood and energetic flow, and get nutrients to the area, the quicker the blockage is opened—or collaterals may form around it. "Blood flows where energy goes", is another slogan of the healing business.

As time went by under the Doc's protocol, the blind spot became smaller. It kind of just went away, and now, two years later, I have no blind spot. My eye is the same as it always was. "How did you bring the dead cells back, or did you?" I asked.

"When there is an infarction, a few cells may die, but the area around it is merely stunned—in shock. If you can restore the blood flow quickly enough, the stunned tissue can resume its normal life."

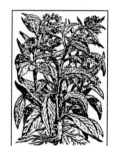
Comfrey plant

"But in addition to acupuncture, you also gave me herbs and several trips into the hyperbaric tank."

"Exactly...! Hyperbaric oxygen is great for these stunned events. Nutrients like lutein and alpha lipoic acid nourish specific neural cells, and help carry out the trash like damaged cell walls. Euphrasia, which is also called Eye Bright is an herb that is specific for enhancing eye health. It's amazing how these little herbal plants know how to help promote health in animals and humans. Why they would want to be symbiotic with animals is beyond my understanding, but they do evidently want to help."

"*Comfrey* is good for cuts and abrasions." The Doc held up a plastic bag of dried leaves. "Put a leaf right on the cut and bandage it. Comfrey contains *allantoin*, which has been clinically shown to promote tissue growth.

"*White Willow Bark* (salix alba) is a natural pain killer and fever reducer." He showed me a pouch of shredded inner bark. "American Indians first used this stuff. They brewed it into a tea. It contains natural salicylic acid, which is what aspirin is made from; but white willow bark won't ruin your stomach lining like synthetic aspirin does."

He pointed to the leaves in two other compartments. "*Spearmint* and *peppermint*." he said. "Good for stomach upset. You can either make a

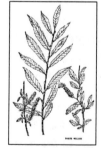
White Willow sapling— stripping outer bark

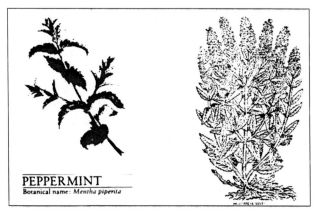

Spearmint and Peppermint

tea, or chew on the leaves if making tea is inconvenient.

"I have two kinds of *Moxa* in the kit," he said. "This normal stick moxa for burning, and this is raw moxa (mugwort)." He held up a wad of brownish cotton. "This stuff is great," he exclaimed. "I saw a guy who had almost cut his thumb off with a fish knife. He came to Dr. Ju to get treated . Dr. Ju grabbed a clump of this furry raw moxa and taped it in place real tightly around the guy's thumb. It's non-poisonous and doesn't cause infection, but you *must* keep it *dry* for ten days after the bandage is in place, or it gets moldy and then you do have infection problems.

"After ten days, the patient came back. Dr. Ju took the bandage off and there was barely even a scar on the guy's thumb. It had been a horrible gash to start with. The fibers of raw moxa knit into a wound and cause it to heal very cleanly."

"How did he keep it dry for ten days…?" I asked.

"What…?" the Doc asked.

"I always get bandages wet. Didn't he take a shower or wash his hands for ten days?"

"How would I know?" he laughed. "The guy didn't want his thumb to fall off. I guess that made him take some special precautions."

"Probably," I said.

"Here's another first aid trick with stick moxa or a burning cigarette," the Doc said. "It's for *nosebleed*.

"If somebody accidentally bonks you on the

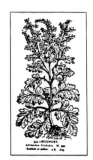

Mugwort plant and fibers

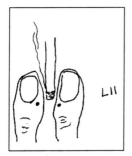

Lighted cigarette and both thumbs, nail side up

nose and it starts to bleed, light a cigarette or a moxa stick or even a stick of incense. Hold it a half inch away from both thumb points at once. To do this you need to hold the thumbs together, and hold the cigarette in your lips."

"Hold the cigarette a quarter inch away from the thumb points until the nose stops bleeding, which should be right away. A cold towel or an ice bag placed over the bridge of the nose also stops bleeding by constricting the blood vessels, but it's not as effective as heat at the thumb points."

*

"How are your goldfish doing..?" I asked. The Doc is fond of koi and keeps a few in a little pond he built in his back yard. Koi lovers are a bit startled to have their prizes referred to as goldfish.

We walked outside to survey the pond. "The main focus of herbs," he reflected, "is not on the energetic level, but on the gross physical level. Herbs are tissue cleaners and purifiers, and tissue builders. That's not to say they don't have an energetic function, but I use them mostly for rough cleaning and large body dysfunctions, not for fine tuning.

"To clean the body internally I use *Saffron* as a diuretic.

Psyllium (Plantago psyllium) is a good bowel cleanser and solves many constipation issues.

Chaparral for lymphatic drainage.

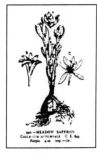

Saffron plant

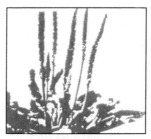

Psyllium plant

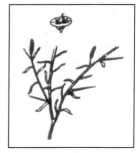

Chaparral bush and leaves

Chapter Fourteen

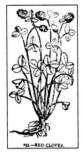
Red Clover plant

Red Clover is an excellent blood purifier."

"Most of these herbs can be purchased at the health food store, but it's a good idea to know what the plant looks like. You could even grow an herb garden in very little space, even on an apartment balcony. Red Clover is often seen growing wild and it's easy to pick out the fuchsia-pink blossoms"

"What was that story about your dad and the car accident?" I asked with one of my famous non-sequiturs, "Wasn't that connected to an herbal cure?"

"My dad was involved in a bad freeway crash while I was still a graduate student at UCLA," the Doc said. "The steering wheel hit him in the chest, partially crushing the ribs against his lungs. Mom called me at Dr. Ju's apartment, saying Dad was lying in bed in terrible pain. He can't even breathe. Please come right away.

"Even before I had finished talking to her, Dr. Ju was writing out a prescription in Chinese for the Chinese herbalist down the street. "Make a tea," Dr. Ju told me. "A big jar. Every day give father some."

"I got the prescription package wrapped in white paper from the herbalist and took it to my parents' house so Mom could boil it into tea. But when I opened the package on the kitchen counter, I knew Dad wouldn't drink it. No way. Several of the ingredients were dried bugs.

"Mom boiled the concoction for the correct amount of time. It smelled up the kitchen, so we moved it to the back porch to cool. We decided not to tell Dad anything about what was in it.

"Dr. Ju sent you this tea to drink," Mom told him.

"It was hard for Dad to move, but he drank a few sips, made a face at the taste, then drank a few more swallows. Immediately, the pain relaxed and he felt better. Two hours later, he started coughing and the chest pain returned. Mom brought another glass of tea and the pain subsided.

"He stayed in bed for a week, then he got up. Eventually, he was totally cured by drinking the herbal tea. Dad was not into esotericism or any alternative medicine, at all. He was a hydraulic engineer and could fix anything."

*

Dr. Ju's Journal—29—Late summer, 1973

Oh, well, I suppose you could say it was my fault. I know, we signed the agreement not to treat outside of the Clinic, but why did the blankity-blank Fresno cops decide to raid the motel where I was treating patients like they never did before? Was it a whim, or did somebody snitch me out? I think about that very often. And now everyone acts like I have committed an outrage because I helped some sick people in exchange for a bit of their money—as I have been doing for thirty years. Especially the Great White Fathers at UCLA. They think it is a sacrilege to help somebody. And doubly so if the sick are poor people and don't have insurance.

Don't get worked up, I tell myself. It is karma. Karma like the rest of it has been. I am not made for the spotlight and so the spotlight gets rid of me when it comes on.

I know I must be starting to repeat myself. It would be far superior to let this go. Maybe move out to Las Vegas or even Tahiti. Why not? But I can't. My mind snaps back like an India rubber string is attached to it. Not good to keep replaying the event, but Fresno cops just don't care about what an old Chinaman does. They never cared before. I was never even visible before. Why am I now? Who told them to have eyes?

These Medical Fathers seem very secure in their medical association, but under the surface are they trembling? Why would that be? No, seriously. Do they really think that acupuncture will take away their fancy car? Or even if they do think that, they could learn acupuncture to augment their practice. Already a few of my students are getting quite skillful, and they have only been at it three or four years.

*

"What happened the time Dr. Ju got arrested?" I asked, still watching the furtive little koi. Dr. Ju Gim Shek had been arrested while working on the UCLA Acupuncture Project for treating patients outside the structure of UCLA without a license. Of course, no one had a license then, and since Dr. Ju was virtually donating his time at UCLA, he felt called upon to earn enough money to feed his family. "How did that arrest go down?" I asked. "To me, treating with acupuncture is a fairly quiet occupation. Why did the Fresno sheriff zone in on him?"

Kathleen, the Doc's wife, answered from the kitchen doorway. "Dr. Ju liked to make a party out of a treatment session," she laughed. "Group sessions were actually how he preferred to work. After a lecture, lots of people were eager to get cured. He'd invite them all to his motel room. He was an amazing guy, and really did help a lot of people; but his sessions got pretty noisy sometimes. I guess that's what happened in Fresno. The police must have thought something very strange was going on." She laughed again. "All those people with needles stuck in them. Of course, it wasn't very funny to us at the time."

"Dr. Ju had technically broken the law," the Doc continued, "that we had written and helped get passed by the California Legislature so that we could open the Clinic at UCLA. Because of the law, it was legal to treat patients in a medical school under an MD's supervision, and illegal to work outside of that structure. Since it became public knowledge that he had broken that law, UCLA felt that he could not represent them in our program that was the first in the country and very open to public scrutiny so they felt compelled to dismiss him from the program. He was quite upset about that decision, but that was what was decided.

"A few years later," the Doc said, "when the Acupuncture Licensing Laws were passed, he was licensed with the rest of us and all was forgiven, but I know it was hard on him. He was an excellent acupuncturist. It was never a question of that. There simply were no licenses for anyone, and we had made ourselves visible at UCLA. And we were having good success with the treatments."

"Being arrested must have been pretty embarrassing for him," I mused. "It doesn't really seem fair."

"It was awful," the Doc said, like he was still in pain over the incident. "The Department of Consumer Affairs officials brought some cops to the UCLA Clinic the next day and took him away in handcuffs. It was a terrible scene, this old respectable Chinese man in handcuffs. Unbelievable."

"This was just several weeks after we had opened the Clinic. As a result, I was left as the only acupuncturist at the Clinic. I treated all the patients, all day long, until Dr. So arrived from Hong Kong six months later. It was a lot of work, and very disruptive to our long term plan." Kathleen nodded agreement.

"What happened then?" I asked.

"He kept treating. That was his life, doing the Doctor, and eventually he moved to Taiwan and semi-retirement," the Doc said. "He was always a great guy, and was vitally important to acupuncture in the United States, and of course, to all of us, his students. I've always felt bad about the shabby way the authorities treated him. Maybe history will correct that injustice. If we hadn't met him in Chinatown, there would be no acupuncture movement here, or at least, not the way it developed."

Chapter Fifteen

First Aid Massage

"Do you think massaging the acupuncture points is as effective as using needles?" I asked Dr. Rosenblatt.

"Of course not," he laughed, "but people don't carry needles around with them. So for first aid, massaging the points is a thousand times better than nothing. Most times it's enough to get you through a crisis.

"Suppose you're doing Tai Chi or playing tennis and you get a bad cramp in your calf (or anywhere in the body). The point to massage is Liver 2 or 3. Liver 3 is better. Use deep twisting pressure with a knuckle or fingertip, like you're screwing in a screw. Massage the point on the side where the cramp occurs. This is a general rule: use the point on the side of the body where the pain is. Liver 3 gives very quick relief.

"You're not trying to hurt the person's foot, but you do need enough pressure to stimulate the energy flow."

"Actually, I got interested in the massage techniques during sword classes in Tai Chi. Somebody was always getting bonked with a wooden sword, and most of the time it was me. These massage points would also be extremely useful in any contact sport like football, basketball or lacrosse.

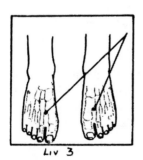

"For instance, a good hit with a lacrosse stick or a hockey stick could easily result in internal injury. It's obvious that this is also a danger in karate and the martial arts. In the event that you think internal hemorrhage is occurring use deep

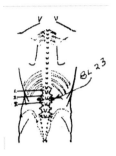

massage with a twisting knuckle at Bladder point 23.

"Also the homeopathic remedy *Arnica* is very useful for injuries of this type. Arnica mobilizes the body's reparative mechanism against injury and trauma. It's from a little plant named Arnica Montana that likes to repair soft tissue in animals. It can be taken internally and/or used as a gel directly on a bruise or sore muscle. Don't use the gel on an open wound.

"Now and then a guy takes a shot to the testicles. A baseball catcher might block three or four bouncing pitches with his scrotum during the course of most seasons. Occasionally a girlfriend or wife might knee a guy in the testicles. It does happen. A low blow in boxing. The point to massage is Kidney Point 2, located halfway up the inside of the foot.

"Deep knuckle on this point will soothe the intense pain. It might even make a guy feel like he'll live. If kneading the point doesn't work, try a percussive massage (a series of quick knuckle hits) on K-2."

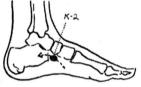

"If an athlete gets the wind knocked out of him by a football helmet in the pit of the stomach and doesn't start breathing easily after a minute or two, use a gentle fingertip massage on Conception Vessel 15, which is located right on the solar plexus. This point is good for any suffocation or difficulty in breathing.

"Coincidentally, CV-15 is also the exact point used for the Heimlich maneuver in CPR first aid for choking on a foreign object in the windpipe.

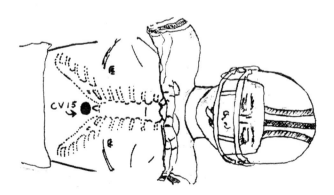

*

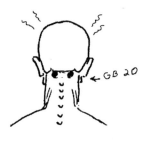

"Headaches occur to most of us now and then. Often they're accompanied by congestion of the blood vessels in the head. Fingertip massage at these two points directly under the base of the skull (Gall Bladder 20) relieves headache at the top and back of the head. It also aids in stopping nose bleed, if you don't have a cigarette handy for the thumb points." (See Chapter 15)

"Also for headache, the point located at the junction of the thumb and forefinger (Large Intestine 4) is quite useful, especially for frontal headache. This point can be massaged by the thumb of the other hand. Massaging LI-4 releases a natural anti-histamine which stops the headache pain.

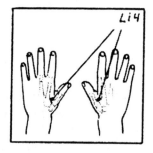

"In the case of extreme physical exhaustion, such as being caught in a snow storm while rock climbing, or using up all your electrolytes in a volleyball championship, apply finger pressure at Governor Vessel 4, which is located under the second lumbar vertebra (lower spine) about an inch above a line joining the hip bones.

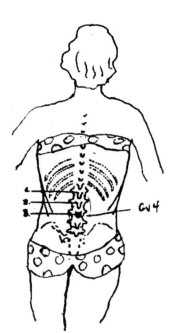

"This point is also good for mental exhaustion, which could occur if a girlfriend leaves the country and you spend too long wondering why. Or if you can't figure out the print command on your new computer."

"To relieve pain anywhere in the body (unless you know the specific point) use gentle massage at Bladder Point 60, behind the ankle bone on the outside of the foot.

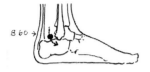

"A little pain is generally experienced at this point, as if it were a receptacle for other pain. Massaging it relieves the ankle pain and helps alleviate any larger source of pain."

"To calm the heart if it malfunctions (palpitations, heart attack) or to calm the spirit, massage Heart Point 7 by using thumb pressure. This is a major relaxation point, located in the crevice medial to the radial bone in the corner of the palm down from the little finger

"Old Chinese grandfathers walk around their gardens with both hands hidden in their sleeves. Inside the sleeve, they are rubbing H-7 on one wrist against H-7 of the other wrist in a swiveling motion, to tonify the heart and calm the spirit."

Several years ago, I was working on a community pottery project to make tiles for a reflecting pool down in Chinatown. The Doc and Elliot Green were on the six person team. We were quite arty during that period. Elliot, a progressive, holistic dentist was in one of the original groups of Dr. Ju's acupuncture students. In any case, I bent over to pick up a box of tiles, something I had done thousands of times in my life with boxes of books and other heavy boxes, but this time something popped in my lower back.

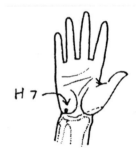

Oh, shoot, I said to myself. I imagined I could feel the bones of my backbone grinding against each other as I tried to stand up. The room went progressively blacker and I passed out cold and fell over. Luckily, Elliot was right there, and caught me. That was very lucky in itself, but he also knew about Conception Vessel 28, in the middle of the cleft in the upper lip.

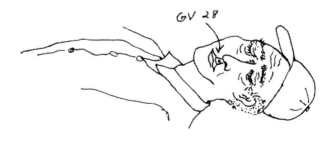

I was out like a light on the dusty concrete floor when he stuck his finger nail in the point in my upper lip. I felt the "finger needle" on my lip and my eyes popped open to see Elliot looking concerned. "I must have passed out," I said to Elliot. "I think my back is broken."

"I doubt it," he said, and he was right. But there were some torn ligaments that took two weeks to heal and hurt like heck.

Dr. Ju's Journal—30—Autumn, 1973

I really loved to watch Bill and the Chairman practice Tai Chi Ch'aun. It reminded me of my own student days. Half the people in Canton did Tai Chi every morning, including the monks at my monastery. Well, maybe not half— Canton has a lot of people.

Chinese people like to do Tai Chi very early, right after dawn. There is a lot of work to accomplish in a Chinese person's day. No time for Tai Chi if he waits for mid-morning. But Bill and the Chairman, and some of the other students, made use of the time before my lecture to practice. Who can fault that? Maybe it kept them from nodding off. I still can't go back to Canton, but here I am in Taiwan visiting my uncle, and treating a few patients from his social club. I love Taiwan. It feels like the old China, which of course it is. The old ways and sensibilities that are now missing on the Mainland came here when the people fled Mao. And, of course, they do Tai Chi early in the morning, almost at dawn.

* * *

Chapter Sixteen

Riding the Tiger

"Tell me about how you guys got acupuncture to be legalized," I said.

"When you jump on a tiger's back, you better hold on tight," the Doc said, with a wry grin. He meant that legalization was like a tiger ride. Once you climb on, you better have a tight grip on a handful of fur or you'll be eaten alive.

"Our first attempt to organize acupuncture teaching and training was the development of the Institute of Taoist Studies in 1970. Bill Prensky and I organized this as a teaching program build around Dr. Ju. Under this organization we trained several dozen practitioners of Chinese Medicine. We gave dozens of presentations and seminars mainly to medical doctors throughout the US.

"But later we sought to expand our focus. Bill Prensky, David Bresler and I had a larger game plan," the Doc said. "That's why the three of us formed the National Acupuncture Association in 1971. Our plan was to change the outlook of American medicine. The first step toward that end was to get our primary treatment method, acupuncture, legalized.

"Bill, David and I were post-graduate laboratory partners at the Psychology Department at UCLA. We were doing experiments on brain/body chemistry and especially on the mechanisms of pain. Through our Tai Chi Chuan instructor, Marshall Ho'o, we met a noted Chinese acupuncturist named Dr. Ju, Gim Shek, (who we mistakenly at first, then affectionately later called Dr. Kim) who was treating patients in Chinatown. We were pretty intense in those early days, and we got really keen on the idea of learning acupuncture. By keen I mean, we hounded Dr. Ju night and day to let us watch him treat patients, and cajoled him into setting up a classroom situation so that we could learn the principles and theories of Chinese medicine, which simply weren't available in English. He thought we should be taught the basic material in a formal classroom setting. And we worked with him in his office in an apprenticeship setting.

"Dr. Ju was a wonderful old guy, who took the time to teach us, primarily because we wanted to learn so badly. We pulled in a few of our friends who were also interested to form his formal classroom setting. I guess there were about fifteen of us at those lectures. Marshall Ho'o, by the way, translated all of the talks, because Dr. Ju was far from fluent in English. Marshall was an excellent communicator. Some of the classes we held around tables in Marshall's Tai Chi studio. Between the two of them, we learned a lot about Oriental ways. Acupuncture in this country owes them a large debt.

"After a time when we had learned some of the fundamentals, Kathleen and I, were selected by Dr. Ju to accompany him to Hong Kong. There we studied at The Hong Kong Acupuncture College with Dr. James Tin Yau So (his name in Chinese is So Tin Yau), who founded the college in 1939. Dr. So spoke English well, was very verbal, and an excellent teacher. After we finished our studies in Hong Kong, and I was running the Clinic at UCLA,

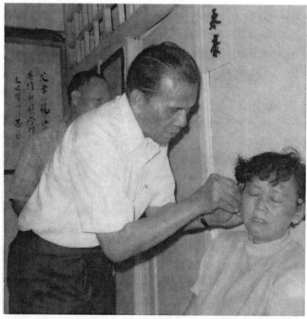

Dr. So treating a patient at the Hong Kong Acupuncture College

Dr. So came to Los Angeles to work in the Clinic. He lived at our house and continued our training on a daily basis. As an aside he was a very accomplished cook and created wonderful Chinese feasts every night.

"When our years at the UCLA Clinic were completed, he and Kathleen and I moved to Boston, where we founded several acupuncture clinics. Here we also founded the James/Stevens Acupuncture College. This was the first acupuncture teaching program in the US. It was originally set up and run in my Tai Chi studio in Boston.

"Dr. So continued to run the college after Kathleen and I came back to Los Angeles. Later the college changed its name and is known today as the New England School of Oriental Medicine. His book, *The Book of Acupuncture Points*, which we began together when he lived with us in Los Angeles, is Volume One of a complete course in acupuncture; it is still in print and is still a very good text. Dr. So insisted that I write the introduction for the book.

"Getting back to the legislation of acupuncture, before there were any acupuncture laws in America, we *could* practice. Everyone considered acupuncture to be a sound medical practice simply because it has such a long history, but there was no license per se. We were in a grey area of medical legality. The obvious place to start was to put a small spot light on acupuncture, and to get the medical establishment to accept it."

"So you, Bill Prensky, and David Bresler sat down one day and decided there had to be some laws?"

"Yes, we went to State Senator Gordon Duffy. Bill had a lawyer friend named Bob Cogan, who knew him. Senator Duffy was a member of the State Committee on Health and Welfare. We convinced him that it was important to have a new way of treating disease; one that could grow out of the Chinese community, which is politically powerful in some areas of California. This was right after President Nixon went to China, so acupuncture was in the news. And here we were in California, the most western state facing China, the perfect place to introduce Chinese medicine.

"Senator Duffy held a series of open hearings on acupuncture. Then he hammered out the first bill, which said that acupuncture could be practiced in a medical school under MD supervision."

"Who testified at the hearings?"

"People like Dr. James Y.P. Chen and other Asian MDs who knew acupuncture. Prensky, Bresler and I, from the National Acupuncture Association, as well as being graduate students at UCLA also made a presentation. We urged the committee to set up a pilot program at a medical school, so the State could take a look at acupuncture in a controlled situation. Now, who could argue with that? There was hardly any opposition. The doctors, of course, loved it. It was under their supervision. The UCLA Acupuncture Project was born in those committee meetings."

"Our game plan was *not* to set up acupuncture in a small, isolated community away from medicine, much like the chiropractic profession had done. The chiropractors got their licensing law passed in 1924 by getting an initiative put on the ballot and having the people vote. They have their own Board of Licensing. We always considered that "The Chiropractic Mistake."

"Our plan was the opposite. We forced the Medical Board to recognize us, in fact we established ourselves right in the middle of the medical community at UCLA Medical School. If you run away and set up your own program, you get isolated."

"What was wrong with the chiropractic method?" I asked.

"The only mistake was a political one. The Medical Board of California and the AMA isolated them. Chiropractors aren't allowed into hospitals. They can't get on staff at any medical schools. They aren't considered for research projects. The AMA won't even talk to them. "You have your own Medical Board. Fine. Just stay there. We'll ignore you."

"We had a different political idea, which was to move into the middle of medicine and set up a tent. Then we'd force the Medical Board to license us."

"But you were inside of medicine already, being at UCLA," I said. "You knew some of the ropes, at least."

"Right. We were inside the medical institution. And we always played the good guy role. We never tried to antagonize the MDs. Our stance was: "Oh, sure, let them supervise us. Sure." We even volunteered our time. I treated patients nine months at the UCLA Clinic for free.

"The National Acupuncture Association started and managed the whole Acupuncture Project for UCLA. We convinced Dr. John Dillon, who was the head of the Department of Anesthesiology. We told him we'd organize the Clinic. We'd staff it. We'd run it. We'd run it on a donation basis, and it wouldn't cost UCLA a penny. In fact, we'd even find the space. Space is the big premium at UCLA. Power equates with how much square footage you control, even more than on the size of your budget. We talked the Psychology Department into donating the space for the Clinic."

"Why would the Psych Department want to give you space?" I asked.

"They wanted to be involved in the project. Bresler and I were doing our graduate work there. We knew where the empty space was. Prensky had left the Psychology Department by then to devote all his time to lobbying for acupuncture; but anyway, we took over the second floor student lounge, which was space that nobody ever used."

"We haven't mentioned David Bresler much in the book," I mused, "but he was pretty important, wasn't he…?"

"David had the best academic credentials of us all. In the early days of the Project, he needed to take a vacation to finish his doctorate. 'You carry the ball for a while," he said to me. "Later on, after I complete my degree, I'll carry it and help you finish your degree.' And a couple of years later, he did."

"What's he doing now?" I asked.

"He's giving seminars on various pain control techniques. One of the techniques he has adapted to pain control is *guided imagery*, where a person imagines himself to be relaxed and not in pain. David studied with Dr. Ju when we all did, and he still uses acupuncture for pain control.

"Anyway, I was managing the Clinic. David was the liaison between the Clinic, which was staffed by the National Acupuncture Association, and the UCLA Medical School. He was the Project Director. I was the Clinic Director. The Clinic had the Medical School all around it. I ran the day to day operations. I was the perfect person, as a practitioner, to run the Clinic, because I had graduated from Hong Kong Acupuncture College."

"Because you really did know more acupuncture?"

"I guess so. I suppose you'd say I was always the leader of the acupuncture treatment program. It broke down neatly. Because David had the best academic credentials at the time, he was always the research and academic liaison person. I always knew the most acupuncture, so I was main practitioner and clinic supervisor. And Bill was the best political organizer I've ever seen. He was the political person. He ran the legal and political maneuvering. His responsibility was the outside community. It was a team that fit together very well."

"How did Prensky get his political expertise?"

"For many years, Bill was one of the directors of the LA Free Clinic in Hollywood."

"Is that right?" I exclaimed. "That was a big deal in the sixties. Did he get that job because of acupuncture?"

"No, before acupuncture. He was a psychology graduate student in the Psychology Department at UCLA when I met him. He ran the psychological counseling service at the Free Clinic. At one point, he ran the whole Free Clinic. It was a very big project, actually.

"Bill gravitated to new age politics," the Doc continued. "He was involved in leading the only hunger strike at UCLA to protest against the Viet Nam War. He spoke in front of the entire student body. We had a tent city on the Commons. Bill was one of the leaders on the UCLA campus. He was a good speaker and a bright guy. Really the guy was a brilliant political organizer. And Bresler was the same way in the area of research and academia. They both were really bright. Super."

"So without the trio, acupuncture legislation might not have worked out?"

"I don't think it would have," the Doc added, "We were all devoted to the expansion, and development of acupuncture as a medical profession in the US. As a group we worked on the political and legal establishment. We also did the research to create the scientific validity of acupuncture from a Western perspective. And we also developed the early practitioner training and protocols."

"Having run the Clinic must have given you an advantage when you testified for the new bill to fully legalize acupuncture?"

"Yes, the UCLA Clinic did help us politically because it was connected to the medical school. We had some clout at last, because we had an effective track record. We treated thousands of patients at UCLA at the Medical School under doctor supervision," he said. "We have case studies with doctors looking at the patients before and after treatment that attest to the results."

"You had staff to keep records…?"

"Of course, we had too. The paper work was enormous, and we were busy trying to get people well. The budget for staff was very thin, so we didn't have many. I was on the run with patients from morning until night. I'd walk into the Clinic every morning and patients would be lined up around the corner. I'm not kidding! They'd be crying at me to treat them…!"

"How many…? Twenty or thirty?"

"At least. Some days I'd treat forty or fifty people. By afternoon on extremely busy days, I'd be so tired, I thought I'd have to run out of the place screaming."

"How many patients are you treating now?" I asked.

"Oh, it can go up to twenty or thirty. But I'm so much more experienced, and my facilities are much, much better. UCLA was scrounge time. At my office, I'm able to control what I do. MDs aren't telling me who to treat, and giving suggestions. At that time we didn't have any money to pay MDs for the Project, so we had helpful volunteers. We were grateful for their help, of course, but suggestions can take up a lot of time.

"As I was saying, the patients would literally be lined up. Remember, there wasn't anywhere else to go for legal acupuncture. Every sick person in the world was there."

"Were these hippies, like at the Free Clinic?" I asked, supposing that's exactly who it would have been in the Sixties.

"Hippies weren't sick," the Doc said. "They had drug problems."

"Hippies got sick like everyone else," I rejoined.

"Hippies had colds. We were treating sick people…! Chronic pain. Multiple sclerosis. People with paralyzed limbs. Terminal cancer."

"Oh. These were people coming as a last resort?"

"Yes. That's what acupuncture was treating. Remember we were in the middle of the UCLA Medical Center. We were getting referrals from the rest of the hospital. Who do you think they were going to send us, people who walked in off the street with a cold? No. 'Let's send this problem case to those acupuncture bozos. See if they can do something. Send the guy still suffering in pain after three spine operations. Get him over there. Let's see what you boys can do. They think they're so hot.'"

I found that amusing. I laughed.

"You think I'm kidding, but that's exactly the way it was."

"So the real walking wounded were waiting in the Clinic hallway every day?"

"Correct. UCLA in general gets all the worst kinds of ailments. If you have something weird, you go there. In private practice, you might treat one or two seriously ill patients a day."

"I always assumed you treated students at the Project Clinic," I said.

"No, hardly ever. I mean, students could get in to see us, but UCLA is one of the biggest research hospitals in the world. If you've gone everywhere else, you end up at UCLA. It's like going to the Mayo Clinic. We treated many prominent and well-known people in the Hollywood community as well as the business and sports worlds"

"So it *was* good for acupuncture to be there. I mean, politically…?" I was having a difficult time getting that through my head. I hadn't realized that UCLA was so important.

"Sure. Excellent," the Doc said. "But what we wanted next was to get acupuncture out of the medical schools. We wanted our own license.

"George Mosconi was a State Senator before he became Mayor of San

Francisco. The Asian community in San Francisco offered him a deal. If he would sponsor licensing of Chinese medicine, they would support him in the Mayoral race. That's a lot of votes in the Bay Area, so he called us in to testify. "Call in the boys from UCLA." So we testified again, since freer more available acupuncture was what we wanted, too. "Yes, acupuncture is safe," we said to the State Senators. "It's effective. It can be regulated. Let's get it out of the medical schools. Sure, we'll have doctor supervision. Give us a license now, and we'll only treat patients who are diagnosed and referred by MDs." So we got what we wanted, it moved the profession of acupuncture closer to our intended goal of full independent licensure, and George Mosconi got elected Mayor of San Francisco.

"We set up that bill so that the Allied Health Division of the California State Medical Board would license acupuncture. Then we formed an advisory committee of acupuncturists to advise the Allied Health Division. Acupuncture didn't even have its own board in the beginning, but the advisory committee eventually became the Acupuncture Board, as it is now."

"Sounds like a real organization," I said.

"We were high powered during those years. And then, of course, we started branching out. Other states came to us when they were getting ready to license acupuncture. We went to Nevada when they were doing licensing. When Oregon was passing their law, we testified. Bill and I set up the entire licensing program and organized the original Oregon State Acupuncture Committee. In fact, because of the Oregon licensing program, I received license number 8, and became the first Westerner licensed in the US"

"The Chinese community in all these places wanted licensing?" I asked.

"Yes."

"So they pushed for it, and you came to assist?"

"We provided the backup. They could talk about thousands of years in China. But we could talk about UCLA, in this country, treating Americans. Not something over there, but right here in a medical school. We had interviews with the Governor of Nevada. Prensky, Dr. Ju and I were introduced on the floor of the Nevada State Senate. That's a big honor. We were a major force behind the licensing in Nevada. And a major force behind and in front of the Oregon Bill, since there wasn't much of a Chinese community in Oregon."

"Legislators liked to talk to you because you could speak English?" I asked.

"Sure, but we could speak scientific jargon, too. We could look up studies. 'Here it is, sir, in this scientific journal.' Naturally, that made acupuncture more comprehensible."

Dr. Ju's Journal—31—Winter, 1973

It was a great honor to be introduced on the floor of the Oregon State Legislature, and then a month later we did it again in Nevada. Carson City is a far cry from Las Vegas. Who would think the capitol would be in a tiny town like that. But it is, so what can one do? They have a few casinos.

Bill and the Chairman were superb in their new suits and fresh haircuts. Very much the young doctors with the horizons to conquer. They explained things about Chinese medicine to the legislators on several occasions that even I had never thought about. The American mind can be very interesting when not consumed with selfish aims.

The speed at which this medicine is being accepted is astonishing. A blink of the eyes ago, I was treating only Chinese patients in my Chinatown office, taking care of my family in that way, but very unknown to the main community of Los Angeles, or America. Now, thanks to my vision and these boys, I am introduced on the venerable floor of state legislatures as an honored physician, almost with the reverence of an ancestor. We travel to Mexico City, where again I am introduced with great dignity and offered to treat difficult patients. It makes me quite proud and grateful.

Of course, I have had a small, dedicated following in Las Vegas, Nevada for a number of years. I love Las Vegas. There I can wear my cowboy boots day and night. In Vegas, they understand certain elements of the human soul that the rest of America hasn't caught up with. And now they have legalized acupuncture. There is something quite wonderful about that. Legal gambling and legal acupuncture. Very civilized.

*

"Once licensing procedures began, naturally all the real acupuncturists wanted to be in the group licensed. They could either take the examination, or if they had enough years of experience they could qualify under the grandfather clause."

"There was a grandfather clause?"

"Most professions are grandfathered in the beginning. If you had been practicing seven years by 1975, you could be grandfathered. I was grandfathered in California although I did take the licensing exam in Oregon."

"And all the Chinese practitioners were practicing that long?"

"Yes. If they could submit credentials that they'd been practicing long enough. The Chinese were very worried about this. How could they say they'd been practicing, when it was illegal before? They thought they might all be arrested if they submitted their patient list. 'Here, sir, are the people I've treated.' Then, they and the patient would be busted. But California accepted everyone in good faith, and no one was hassled. And they're now licensed. A lot of good people got busted before the law was passed. Grandfathering is like an amnesty to get legalization started. Three to four hundred practitioners got licensed under the grandfather clause. Mainly they were Chinese who had been here for years."

"I suppose the licenses and the State Examination led right into you opening your own acupuncture college?" I asked.

"No, that came later. In the beginning we were training MDs in programs that we set up with Dr. Ju under the banner of the Institute of Taoist Studies. We had a class of doctors who we lectured to at UCLA. MDs can practice any kind of medicine on their current license, so they could practice acupuncture as soon as they learned some. One of the functions of the National Acupuncture Association was to train people in acupuncture. But we finally realized that if we wanted really good acupuncturists, we had to train acupuncturists from the beginning."

"Why didn't you train MDs?"

"Well, they didn't have the right mind set for acupuncture. They were thinking Western all the time. They'd do a little acupuncture, but only a couple of them got good at it. It forced us to realize that if we were going to be a profession, we needed our own professionals out there practicing. So we shifted away from training MDs and decided to train our own specialists. At that point we started thinking about a school of our own."

"The next step," the Doc said, "was to get the Diagnosis and Referral by MD clause dropped from the acupuncture law."

"Obviously, the Chinese practitioners didn't want that clause either."

"No. They wanted it dropped, so they led the fight to have it deleted. We testified before the State Legislature again. 'There hasn't been any problems in the field,' we said. 'Who has been hurt?' Acupuncture still to this day has a very, very low percentage of problems compared to other medical practices. There have been very few malpractice cases against it. Very few. The reason is that acupuncturists are interested in maintaining health and balancing energy. They're not giving drugs, and they're not doing surgery. The worst objection was that we might miss a diagnosis. And it is possible not to catch a cancerous tumor in a very early stage, for instance. But there are a million doctors around. We're not out in the wilderness as the only medical personnel. There's no chance that someone doesn't have access to other medical help. So the legislature finally agreed with us and dropped the Diagnosis and Referral clause from the law.

"Acupuncturists, of course, have their own special interests. We worked hard to pass an insurance bill in 1984, so we could be reimbursed by the insurance companies. The idea of treating patients in a non-invasive way (no drugs or surgery) should be very appealing to insurance companies."

"Also acupuncturists don't charge as much as other doctors," I added.

"Right. It saves money. Saves the insurance companies money, saves the public money. There are no fees for extensive testing, and of course, surgery costs a fortune."

"Are the insurance companies on your side? I'd think they would be."

"They are, sort of. But because they're tied in with the MDs and the pharmaceutical companies, it's hard for them to divorce their thought from the medical establishment."

"Because...?"

"Well, they don't really want to pay for another service. Acupuncture is just one more thing, and they don't particularly want to cover it."

"Even though it saves them money?"

"It would save them money, but every additional service that they cover is money out of their pocket. They think that if they don't cover acupuncture, the people will go to an MD. You have insurance, would you go to an MD?" he asked me.

"Not often," I replied.

"Right. You'd learn to live with the pain. The MD would say, "I'm sorry, there's nothing I can do for your back. You'll have to live with it." So the insurance company wouldn't have to pay for you to live with it."

"If you don't count the traction, and the month in a hospital and the doctor's fee."

"They see it as an additional medical treatment that people would use. The theory is that people who aren't going to get surgery, don't get surgery. That theory is only partly true, because some people who are considering surgery will try something else first. Acupuncture. And they'll be helped. And that would save the insurance company a lot of money."

"Has it ever occurred to you," I asked the Doc, "that when this book comes out you'll be getting calls from all over the country to treat weird things?"

"Sure. But I already do. The thing that strikes me is that we're seeing a miracle. Acupuncture is licensed as a primary health care profession in California and many other states. I tell all my entering students that a miracle has happened. The fact that acupuncture, which relies on treating the body's energy level and manipulating energy with needles, is now licensed in America is a major phenomenon, a true miracle. In only thirty years, we took acupuncture from unknown to fully licensed and well known."

"It wasn't totally unknown to the Chinese," I observed.

"Of course, it was known in the Chinese community, but to the mass of Americans, acupuncture was a foreign word and a foreign concept. I'd never heard of it myself the first time somebody mentioned acupuncture. Never heard the word! And I was a graduate student at UCLA at the time. You can stop almost anyone on the street now, and not only have they heard of it, but they have a firm opinion. We have actually changed medicine! Which was what we intended from the beginning. That was our whole game plan at UCLA. We decided we were going to change the health care delivery system in California, and from there the rest of the country. The change was in viewing medicine as an energetic system.

"We believed that studying the laws of energetic medicine would give new keys to extension of life, and prevention and cure of disease. By looking at the body from another point of view, all these things might be possible. Rather than diagnosing symptoms and effects of disease, which is the approach of Western medicine, we looked for the causes. What is malfunctioning? Is there a short circuit in the energy system? How can we prevent it from short circuiting? Once it has short circuited, what can be done to correct the situation, rather than simply cutting an important organ out.

"So we gave up the idea of training MDs. Real practitioners of this energetic medicine were needed. Energetic medicine doctors to go into the community. We had to have a school where we could train these people from ground zero, to be pioneers. That was the big secret. That's why I opened the California Acupuncture College in Los Angeles. At this same time, Kathleen started teaching classes in Santa Barbara at the Cottage Hospital and at Santa Barbara City College. Her classes dovetailed into the Calfornia Acupuncture College when the accreditation came through.

"I told every incoming class at the College that they're being trained as doctors of energetic medicine. I reminded them again when they graduated. They were stuffed with everything we've learned about Energetics—from acupuncture, to homeopathy, to radionics. Of course, technology will expand with new machines and techniques involving finer electro-magnetic field equipment. The students will be schooled in the energetic principles, and then they'll go out as pioneers—affecting all of medicine. Applying their concepts and understanding to many new situations and conditions. Eventually, when they treat enough patients successfully, we'll reach a critical mass. So many people will be attuned to the idea of Energetics, that Americans will no longer be forced to rely on drugs and surgery. They'll want to look to prevention of illness, early treatment, maintenance—all the things we've been talking about.

"And that, of course, is the reason for this book," the Doc said. "Another attempt to cast this idea into the main stream. How can we get people aware of and interested in a different approach to medicine? We're doing it. People want to be healthy, and their energetic system always strives to be in balance.

"When my colleagues and I were young and dumb we took a ride on the tiger's back. And we were pretty successful at it. We thought we could accomplish great deeds; but naturally, there were certain things we didn't take into account because we didn't know enough. We knew we didn't know enough, but that is the human condition. Since we didn't really meet much resistance, and the time was right for change, we had some success. We were schooled by wonderful teachers who had great foresight. We always realized there was a lot more to know; but the principles are here, and we are still learning."

Dr. Ju's Journal—32—Autumn, 1975

Keeping this journal has become a habit, part of my daily routine. I am feeling old now, well, sort of old. Dr. So Tin Yao, the Hong Kong Professor, is at the UCLA clinic with my former students making medical history, being written up in the medical journals, treating movie stars, while I am here in Hong Kong making a different kind of history. A slower one. My uncle has arranged for me to lecture here and over in Taipei. He has reserved a small ballroom, where afterwards I will treat the peoples' illnesses. This is the way healing is done in a civilized country. Heal the blocked energy, and enjoy the process. Like a healing party. That is the civilized way.

In Hong Kong I can dine several evenings a week with my friends the Tan-ka boat people. The Tan-ka are elegant at face saving, and their food is simple, but extremely excellent. I cannot wear my cowboy boots here, obviously. It would be preposterous to jump into a water taxi in my boots. Tipping myself into the oily waters of Hong Kong harbor would not be a smart thing to do. No, the boots await my return to Las Vegas where my friends are urging me to visit. The acupuncture law is passed in Nevada, as I said. I have been conferred a license. Please come they say, "We eagerly await you."

One day I may go again. Treating sick people is what I do. People everywhere have illness, and I must pay for my expensive habits of eating and breathing. It makes an opportunity to trade—healing for money, which after all is the Taoist way of the doctor. Taoists do not beg with the begging bowl.

Yes, it is my time to go back to the home of my ancestors. It is not so easy living among the barbarians. My mission in America, where I was sent by my Taoist monk teachers so long ago, is accomplished. My students will tend the garden, growing the medicine we have planted from a sacred seed for the benefit of all mankind. All is harmony.

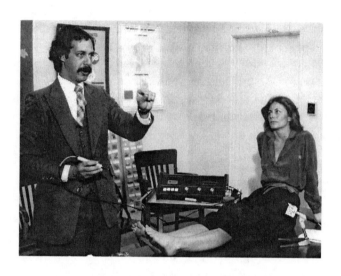

THE END

About the Authors

Steven Rosenblatt was a graduate student in Physiological Psychology at UCLA when he began to train in Acupuncture and Oriental Medicine under Dr. Ju Gim Shek in Los Angeles. After a three year apprenticeship, he went to Hong Kong where they graduated from the Hong Kong Acupuncture College, the first western student of Dr. James Tin Yau So. On his return to Los Angeles, he organized and was the clinical director of the UCLA Acupuncture Research Project in UCLA's Department of Anesthesiology, the first acupuncture clinic in a medical school in the USA.

Dr. Rosenblatt brought Dr. So to this country to work on the UCLA clinic project for several years before moving to Boston where they organized the James-Stevens Acupuncture Center, the first training program in the USA, that grew into today's New England School of Acupunctre.

Returning to Los Angeles, Dr. Rosenblatt established the California Acupuncture College, with branches in Santa Barbara (which later became the Santa Barbara Acupuncture College) and San Diego (which evolved into the Pacific College of Oriental Medicine.

Dr. Rosenblatt was deeply involved in creating a licensure program for Acupuncture. He helped create licensing regulations, speaking and lobbying for legislation in Nevada, Oregon and California. In 1974, he received license number 8 in the State of Oregon, the first Westerner to be licensed to practice Acupuncture in the USA.

Dr. Rosenblatt received his Ph.D. from UCLA for his dissertation, "Electrophysiological Correlates of Acupuncture Points." This was the first doctoral research dissertation on Acupuncture at a major university in the United States.

As president of the California Acupuncture College, Dr. Rosenblatt helped establish several of the national educational and accreditation agencies. This college served as a template to set the cirterions used by the state of California's agencies. He served on the National Accreditation Commission for Schools and Colleges of Oriental Medicine for six years, helping to review and accredit many of the acupuncture and Oriental medicine schools in this country.

After twenty years in the Acupuncture and Oriental Medicine fields, Dr. Rosenblatt went back to medical school and earned an MD degree from St. Georges University. He completed his medical school training in England and went on to do a Family Practice residency at Kaiser Hospital in Riverside, CA.

Dr. Rosenblatt is National Board Certified in Acupuncture. He is licensed as a medical doctor in California and Hawaii. He is residency trained in Family Practice and is currently board certified in Urgent Care Medicine.

Dr. Rosenblatt served on the 1984 Olympics Medical Advisory Team, and on the Advisory Committee of the American Nutraceutical Association. He helped develop and served as the Program Coordinator of Complimentary Medicine Program at Cedars-Sinai Medical Center.

He is the author of many published research articles, and his best selling book "The Starch Blocker Diet" was published by HarperCollins. This book is now selling the paperback edition and has been translated and published in a German language edition.

Dr. Rosenblatt is a nationally recognized leader in the fields of Integrative and Complementary Medicines. He maintains a busy clinical practice combining Family Practice medicine, Acupuncture and Complimentary modalities with offices in West Los Angeles, Van Nuys, Eagle Rock and the Big Island of Hawaii. He is currently on staff at Saint John's Health Center in Santa Monica, CA.

Keith Kirts has written twenty novels, science fiction and detective. Many are available on Amazon, Kindle and at your local bookstore.

CPSIA information can be obtained
at www.ICGtesting.com
Printed in the USA
LVOW12*1820021017
550904LV00013B/267/P

9 781504 364331